The International Library of Bioethics

Volume 88

The *International Library of Bioethics* – formerly known as the International Library of Ethics, Law and the New Medicine comprises volumes with an international and interdisciplinary focus on foundational and applied issues in bioethics. With this renewal of a successful series we aim to meet the challenge of our time: how to direct biotechnology to human and other living things' ends, how to deal with changed values in the areas of religion, society, and culture, and how to formulate a new way of thinking, a new bioethics.

The *International Library of Bioethics* focuses on the role of bioethics against the background of increasing globalization and interdependency of the world's cultures and governments, with mutual influencing occurring throughout the world in all fields. The series will continue to focus on perennial issues of aging, mental health, preventive medicine, medical research issues, end of life, biolaw, and other areas of bioethics, whilst expanding into other current and future topics.

We welcome book proposals representing the broad interest of this series' interdisciplinary and international focus. We especially encourage proposals addressing aspects of changes in biological and medical research and clinical health care, health policy, medical and biotechnology, and other applied ethical areas involving living things, with an emphasis on those interventions and alterations that force us to re-examine foundational issues.

More information about this series at https://link.springer.com/bookseries/16538

Megan A. Allyse · Marsha Michie
Editors

Born Well: Prenatal Genetics and the Future of Having Children

Springer

Editors
Megan A. Allyse
Program in Biomedical Ethics Research
Mayo Clinic
Jacksonville, FL, USA

Marsha Michie
Department of Bioethics
Case Western Reserve University
Cleveland, OH, USA

ISSN 2662-9186 ISSN 2662-9194 (electronic)
The International Library of Bioethics
ISBN 978-3-030-82535-5 ISBN 978-3-030-82536-2 (eBook)
https://doi.org/10.1007/978-3-030-82536-2

This Springer imprint is published by the registered company Springer Nature Switzerland AG
The registered company address is: Gewerbestrasse 11, 6330 Cham, Switzerland

Introduction

The landscape of prenatal screening has changed dramatically since the mid-1980s, when Alfa-Fetoprotein (AFP) and other serum markers were first used as fetal screening protocols. As we enter the third decade of the twenty-first century, we are rapidly moving into a phase of prenatal care in which broad spectrum genetic screening of fetal DNA is becoming routine. Fetal exome and genome sequencing, still largely conducted under research protocols, will almost certainly be integrated into clinical prenatal care within the next few years. At the same time, polygenic risk scores are being offered for assisted reproduction, promising to measure increasingly detailed metrics of which embryo is most likely to result in the "best" child (Treff et al., 2019). The ability to detect mosaicism, HLA type, and key genetic markers of disease presents potential parents with a widening array of choices even before pregnancy begins. And in 2019, the prospect of deliberately altering human embryos to determine certain traits entered the conversation when a Chinese scientist claimed to have used CRISPR-CAS9 technology to alter the genes of several embryos in an effort to confer increased immunity to HIV/AIDS (Allyse et al., 2019). All of these technologies present the potential to improve standards of "health," and indeed to alter the ways in which we define health itself. Despite condemnation of the premature use of germline CRISPR modifications, responses to the potential avoidance of disease through embryo selection have largely been positive. Parents of children with serious hereditary conditions have hailed prenatal screening and preimplantation genetic diagnosis as a means to avoid the suffering associated with conditions such as sickle cell anemia or alpha thalassemia (Hill, Compton, Karunaratna, Lewis, & Chitty, 2014; Farra et al., 2008; Darbari et al., 2018). And certain communities, such as the American Ashkenazi Jewish community, have elevated carrier screening and PGD to a systematic effort to eliminate Tay–Sachs disease in their population (Gross, Pletcher, & Monaghan, 2008). Some scholars have gone so far as to imagine a future in which all pregnancies are not only predicted but planned, with every embryo undergoing scrutiny before it becomes a potential fetus (Greely, 2016).

But as Rayna Rapp detailed in her seminal work on amniocentesis, the ability to learn ever greater amounts of biological information about the developing fetus has both advanced maternal fetal health and created an ever widening set of social and ethical dilemmas about the consequences of that information and how we act on it (Rapp, 1999). At the core of such debates is the question of who should or should not be born and the gatekeepers that make or substantially influence those decisions. As we move into an era in which genetic science, and the choices it makes possible, increasingly shape our offspring, we continue to ask ourselves how far we should go in an effort to give those offspring a "good birth." What does it mean to have a "healthy" child–to ensure our children are born "well"?

The term "eugenics," coined in 1883 by British scientist Francis Galton, translates directly into "good birth" (Galton, 1904) Early eugenicists conceptualized selecting which births went forward as a means of improving health on the grounds that healthy people led to healthy, and thus more virtuous, societies. Thus, public campaigns to encourage prudent selection of spouses and healthy habits for children formed the "positive" arm of the eugenics movement. But the movement also included systemic, State-led programs enacting targeted elimination of certain classes of individuals, typically the poor and racial/ethnic minorities. The California eugenics laws of the early twentieth century, for example, focused on individuals deemed "unfit" or "feeble minded": terms that were frequently weaponized against women of color (Stern et al., 2017). Such programs were prominent in the United States in the 1920s and 30s, and many of the practices commonly attributed to the Third Reich in their pursuit of racial cleansing were inspired by and drawn from United States eugenic policies (Black, 2003). Societies now widely condemn such practices, and rightly so. But as Troy Duster points out, the expanding control that medicine provides over which children are chosen and birthed essentially leads us to a different form of eugenics (Duster, 2003). This "backdoor" to eugenics means that, in a societal context in which power and wealth accrue to those with particular physical characteristics, it is realistic to expect that parents who can choose more valorized physical characteristics will often do so. Those choices not only include being male, tall, and fair-skinned (all of which correlate in the US to higher salary)(Hamstra, 2014) but also the absence of disabling conditions–since people with disabilities face significant social and economic disadvantages.

Prenatal screening and testing technologies are often promoted on the basis of increasing parental autonomy and reproductive liberty. The goal, many claim, is not to promote genetic selection but to aid parental "preparation" and informed choice. But as Duster points out, enlightened self interest does not result in equity unless all other features of the social environment are held constant (Duster, 2003). Individual choices, while reasonable in the context of the social situation in which people are embedded, can, in aggregate, amount to major population-level change. Even when individuals acknowledge that these forces are damaging, few parents would resist making choices that benefit themselves and their potential child. In a society in which there remain significant physical, social, economic, and political disparities, it is reasonable for a responsible parent to select the child most likely to thrive in that society (Hvistendahl, 2011). Does this logic render the selection of embryos unethical or does it suggest that the technology cannot create injustice in a vacuum? Does surveillance technology like prenatal screening and testing create social difference or does it merely allow us to project our existing inequalities and biases into the womb?

Ethical arguments for and against selective pregnancy termination have been debated since the first technologies for prenatal screening and diagnosis appeared on the horizon. In many ways, those underlying ethical arguments have not changed. What is new, as technological possibilities have changed, diversified, and accelerated, are the massively wider social and ethical consequences of these technologies. As these new technologies appear and become broadly available, even routine, a large-scale change in the human phenotype is now more than a science fiction fantasy. And as these possibilities come closer to everyday reality, it is crucial to revisit the ethical and social arguments about prenatal testing and selection from the perspectives of both individual families and whole societies. In the chapters that follow, we will explore these dilemmas from a variety of perspectives. The authors represented here are far from comprehensive. No one volume can encompass the array of perspectives on a set of issues that are arguably relevant to everyone in our society. But the chapters that follow represent a cross section of the debates we are having, and will continue to have, as the practice of prenatal medicine continues to incorporate increasing amounts of technological information.

Part I

We begin with an overview of the current clinical landscape and the ways in which practitioners, who encounter women and families every day, envision their profession moving forward. In Chap. 1, Ruth Farrell, a practicing OB/GYN and bioethicist, offers insight into how the increasing amount of genetic information available during pregnancy may or may not change the practice of obstetric and maternal–fetal medicine and its outcomes. Among the many ethical and societal issues are the everyday decisions families and practitioners make. How much information is too much? When does the volume of genetic information drown out more prosaic, but reliable, measures of health and wellness? These are themes that continue in the following chapter by Wendy Chung, a clinical geneticist, on pediatric medicine and its adaptations to genomic information. Both authors point out that while the clinical translation of genomic technologies has proceeded with a momentum of its own, it remains unclear the extent to which outcomes, both subjectively and objectively measured, will see concrete improvement. With each major advance in prenatal genetic and genomic technologies we return to many of the same issues. Technologies do not pre-determine the ways in which they may be used, though social and ethical ideas about intended uses shape those technologies from the beginning. And as more voices have entered scientific, medical, and ethical conversations about prenatal genomics we have begun to bridge the micro-level debates about the contours of specific technologies with macro-level debates about social uses of genomics. In that middle space lies the individual decision-making of parents and families, guided by individual encounters with healthcare providers; yet these are invisibly shaped by both the technologies themselves and our social understandings of genomics.

Part II

Among the first organized groups to critique prenatal genetic testing were families of people with Down syndrome–not surprisingly, since Down syndrome was one of the first targets of prenatal testing, and remains the lens through which many view both prenatal testing and genetic conditions more generally. The voices of advocates in the Down syndrome community, even today, are particularly prominent and eloquent in debates over prenatal screening. Down syndrome is the most common chromosomal condition in live-born babies, it entails distinctive facial features that are easily recognizable, and it is among the easiest conditions to look for during pregnancy. Down syndrome has been the subject of prenatal testing for over 50 years, and is part of all current prenatal screening and testing protocols. And the very definition of "high-risk" pregnancy due to advanced maternal age is based on the intersection between the procedure-related risk of amniocentesis and the age-related risk of Down syndrome (Kuppermann & Goldberg..., 1999). But the perceived severity of Down syndrome has changed radically over those past fifty years, due primarily to parents' and advocates' insistence on de-institutionalizing and mainstreaming children with Down syndrome. Those social changes account for the meteoric rise in life expectancy for people with Down syndrome, from approximately 20 years in 1970 to over 60 years today (Saul & Meredith, 2016).

Part II explores some ways that people in Down syndrome and other disability communities view prenatal screening and testing and what those perspectives can teach us about expanding into other conditions. In Chap. 3, Mark Leach discusses some parallels between current-day prenatal genetic testing programs and eugenics programs of the past, concluding that these common features could be counteracted by funding models that do not subsidize the tests themselves without also providing funding for genetic counseling and up-to-date information for families. Louise Bryant and Tom Shakespeare, in Chap. 4, review recent empirical research with people with disabilities and their families to highlight disconnects between their lived experience and the more negative information and attitudes toward disabilities conveyed by healthcare providers and policymakers in discourses about prenatal genetic testing. In Chap. 5, Christopher Kaposy builds upon his previous work on the expressivist critique of Down syndrome testing, expanding upon these arguments to address the ever-broadening panels being offered via prenatal cfDNA screening, chromosomal microarrays, and preimplantation genetic diagnosis–along with other prenatal technologies on the horizon such as whole genome sequencing and CRISPR gene modification.

Part III

As multiple technologies of prenatal genetics and genomics have moved from laboratory discovery into clinical innovation and cultural experiences of pregnancy and childbirth, we have grappled with them–individually and as a whole–in philosophy, theology, social science, and the humanities. What is the meaning of genetic health or disability? What cultural, religious, and socioeconomic forces nudge pregnant women and families toward or away from an imperative to know genomic information about their future child? And how do those broader forces shape clinical encounters and decisions that are never, as we imagine, simply "between a woman and her doctor"? Insights from cultural, social, and religious studies can help us understand these encounters and decisions more deeply than as a simple, rational weighing of pros and cons, barriers and facilitators.

We start, in Chap. 6, with "the hypothetical healthy newborn," a theoretical figure that literary, bioethics, and disability studies scholar Rosemarie Garland-Thomson summarizes as "a promise that cannot be kept." As an idealized concept that never matches the necessary imperfection of a real child, Garland-Thomson argues that clinical genetic technologies simultaneously chip away at the ideal of the healthy newborn with diagnostic information and, continually and increasingly, hold out the promise of approaching that ideal through knowledge and treatment. But while potential parents may take advantage of opportunities to know about, treat, and/or terminate their fetus in order to approximate the hypothetical healthy newborn, Garland-Thomson proposes an alternative: to consider the vitality of a distinctive, growing being as a range of human variation to be celebrated and accommodated.

Discussions of prenatal screening in United States discourse inevitably bring up the possibility of pregnancy termination. Indeed, some observers in the Evangelical community have decried all prenatal screening because it suggests, to them, the acceptability of termination based on the findings. For these believers, the fetus in the womb is the future child chosen by God for this family and no medical surveillance should suggest otherwise. While this approach ignores the other clinical and psychosocial value that fetal information may have, it nevertheless has significant adherents, including former Senator Samuel Brownback, a vocal opponent of abortion under any circumstances. One tradition that has engaged with historic opposition to pregnancy termination in a more nuanced way is the Roman Catholic Church. Although Catholicism is by no means the only religious tradition to grapple with prenatal surveillance and disability, we include it here for two reasons. One, institutions run in the Catholic tradition are the fastest growing health systems in the United States, and Catholic outreach around health is prevalent worldwide (Wascher, Hebert, Freedman, & Stulberg, 2018). Secondly, given its long history of concerted scholarship around issues of health and medicine, the Catholic Church has one of the most clearly articulated bioethical traditions of all major religions. In his chapter, Fr. Kevin Fitzgerald explores how the Church's thinking on prenatal information has evolved as technologies have advanced. A historically pro-natalist organization, the Church has struggled to balance the health goals of prenatal screening with concerns about its association with the termination of pregnancies found to be affected by medical conditions. In doing so, the Church has come to reject binary understandings of technologies like prenatal screening and testing as being either supportive of or inimical to health and human thriving. Fitzgerald quotes Pope John Paul II, who said "moral evaluation and scientific research must go hand in hand, and … charity must animate them in a harmonious interdisciplinary whole, marked by unity and distinction." Thus, the Church's duty to the value of human life and protection of the weak supports the potential beneficial applications of surveillance technologies, he notes, so long as their use furthers the goal of human thriving.

However, what human thriving looks and feels like varies significantly between societies, cultures, and individuals lives. In Chap. 8, for instance, we (Michie and Allyse) outline a history of how prenatal technologies have come to be deeply intertwined with social pressures toward womanhood and, in particular, motherhood. Mid-century tropes around the role of women in society, and in particular post-war anxieties about the role of women in the workforce, led to a prevailing philosophy that "a good mother should have no interests of her own." That is, the interests of the fetus and the interests of the good mother should be indistinguishable. As such, whatever the medical system or prevailing wisdom dictates is the correct course of action to advance the health and wellness of the fetus becomes, by definition, the morally correct action for the mother to take. As prenatal testing began in the 1970s, the linkage between responsible motherhood and surveillance of the fetus was strengthened to the point that in some jurisdictions screening became the default.

This trend coincides with, or is perhaps co-produced by, the neoliberal growth of the commensurability of health. Also originating in the 1950s was the idea of indirect cost, which measures the monetary cost to society of ill health or disability in a population. The idea of indirect cost was originally developed in service of the Liberal aim of increasing Federal regulation and supervision of worker and workplace safety, arguing that, because there were economic impacts of worker injuries or deaths the State had a valid interest in reducing them (Rice, Hodgson, & Kopstein, 1985). Similar arguments in the 1970s fueled support for restrictions on tobacco advertising and usage. However, as the shift to neoliberal governance grew, the idea of the economic cost of disability or illness expanded to include congenital conditions. In 1994, Waitzman and co-authors published "Estimates of the Economic Cost of Birth Defects," in which individuals with Down syndrome were framed as posing a lifelong loss to society of productivity and income based on the assumption that they would be a net consumer, not producer, of goods and services (Waitzman, Romano, & Scheffler, 1994). This framing led to the inexorable logic that society had an economic interest in the prevention of births of "unproductive" individuals and brought us full circle to the original aims of eugenics. By 2015, Peter Benn was using Waitzman's estimate of the lifetime cost of a person with Down syndrome to argue that noninvasive genetic screening was more cost effective than serum marker screening. The logic presented was that while genetic testing might be more expensive, it was also more accurate. The lifetime savings of avoiding a child with Down syndrome would thus compensate for the increased cost of testing (Benn et al., 2015).

Part IV

One aspect of prenatal genetic technologies has not changed at all since their inception: that they are continually changing, growing, and becoming ever more precise. So as we consider the ethical, clinical, and social aspects of prenatal testing and selection, we inevitably look toward a future in which these technologies are even more advanced, more pervasive, and more accessible. What lessons can we take from the history of prenatal screening and testing to inform this future and, conversely, what can imagining that future help us illuminate about today's debates?

The last part of this volume begins to address these questions and does so with only a single chapter. In Chap. 9, bioethicist David Wasserman takes current debates about prenatal genetics into a world where it's possible to precisely select the characteristics of one's future child, by creating an imaginatively futuristic version of a parent's guide to what to expect during pregnancy. When it's possible to create a large supply of embryos from a parent's skin cells, and then select the most genetically desirable one of these using whole genome sequencing–and not only possible, but cheap and covered by insurance–the imperative to choose one's most perfect possible offspring may be nearly irresistible. Wasserman takes on the challenge of convincing parents in this imagined future world to resist that imperative, and in so doing he makes an ethical case *for* prenatal testing yet *against* prenatal selection, attempting to ethically separate these two options that have for so long been conjoined in clinical decision-making. His arguments render current debates over prenatal genetics into plain language that, by addressing a hypothetical future, shed considerable light on a contentious present.

Conclusion

The clinical landscape of prenatal screening and testing is evolving rapidly. At time of writing, efforts were underway to mandate universal Medicaid coverage of noninvasive prenatal genetics testing, enable expanded carrier screening in all pregnancies, and increase use of multiplex sequencing in the prenatal space. Private companies now offer polygenic risk evaluation of in vitro embryos to calculate complex disease risk and embryo screening for eye and hair color. Several states have attempted to pass laws banning elective termination on the basis of prenatal determination of sex, race, and Down syndrome status. And yet, the more things change, it seems, the more things stay the same. We are still having crucial, difficult conversations about fundamentals of reproductive rights and freedoms. Who decides the value of a good life and one that is worth living? What is the role of disability in society, and what does disability even mean in the context of medical advancement that have made physical survival more likely but done comparatively little to address social and economic exclusion and discrimination? Every time a new advancement in assisted reproduction is introduced, whether it is preimplantation genetic diagnosis, mitochondrial transfer, or CRISPR repair of single gene mutations, the media abounds with invocations of the spectre of "designer babies." But what is a designer baby and how does it differ from the thousands of ways we have manipulated ourselves and our offspring over the generations? Pundits frequently argue that "the technology is outpacing the ethics" in assisted reproduction. But more often, new technologies change only the terminology, not the ethical calculus. Ultimately, we argue in this volume, it is not technology that ushers in the ethical dilemmas. We must engage with these foundational moral conundra repeatedly, consistently, and in an inclusive arena that involves stakeholders from across the many elements of human society irrevocably bound up in the process and results of reproduction. We hope that the chapters here are a meaningful contribution to that conversation, and will help readers engage with these fascinating questions.

References

Allyse, M., Y. Bombard, R. Isasi, M. Michie, K. Musunuru, and K. E. Ormond. 2019. What do we do now?: Responding to claims of germline gene editing in humans. *Genet Med*, 21(10), 2181–2183.

Benn, P., K.J. Curnow, S. Chapman, S.N. Michalopoulos, J. Hornberger, and M. Rabinowitz. 2015. An Economic Analysis of Cell-Free DNA Non-Invasive Prenatal Testing in the US General Pregnancy Population. *PLoS One*, *10*(7), e0132313.

Black, E. 2003. *War against the weak: Eugenics and America's campaign to create a master race*. Washington, DC: Dialog Press.

Darbari, I., J.E. O'Brien, S.J. Hardy, B. Speller-Brown, L. Thaniel, B. Martin, et al. 2018. Views of parents of children with sickle cell disease on pre-implantation genetic diagnosis. *Pediatric blood & cancer*, *65*(8), e27102.

Duster, T. 2003. *Backdoor to eugenics*. New York: Routledge.

Farra, C., A.H. Nassar, I.M. Usta, P. Salameh, M. Souaid, and J. Awwad. 2008. Acceptance of preimplantation genetic diagnosis for β-thalassemia in Lebanese women with previously affected children. *Prenatal Diagnosis: Published in Affiliation With the International Society for Prenatal Diagnosis*, *28*(9), 828–832.

Galton, F. 1904. Eugenics: Its definition, scope, and aims. *American Journal of Sociology*, *10*(1), 1–25.

Greely, H.T. 2016. *The end of sex and the future of human reproduction*. Cambridge: Harvard University Press.

Gross, S.J., B.A. Pletcher, and K.G. Monaghan. 2008. Carrier screening in individuals of Ashkenazi Jewish descent. *Genetics in Medicine*, *10*(1), 54–56.

Hamstra, M.R W. 2014. 'Big'men: Male leaders' height positively relates to followers' perception of charisma. *Personality and Individual Differences*, *56*, 190–192.

Hill, M., C. Compton, M. Karunaratna, C. Lewis, and L. Chitty. 2014. Client Views and Attitudes to Non-Invasive Prenatal Diagnosis for Sickle Cell Disease, Thalassaemia and Cystic Fibrosis. *J Genet Couns*, 23(6), 1012–1021.

Hvistendahl, M. 2011. *Unnatural selection : choosing boys over girls, and the consequences of a world full of men* (reprint ed.). New York: PublicAffairs.

Kuppermann, M., and Goldberg…, J.D. 1999. Who should be offered prenatal diagnosis? The 35-year-old question. *American Journal of Public Health*, 89(2), 160–163.

Rapp, R. 1999. *Testing women, testing the fetus: The social impact of amniocentesis in America* New York: Routledge.

Rice, D.P., T.A. Hodgson, and A.N. Kopstein. 1985. The economic costs of illness: a replication and update. *Health care financing review*, *7*(1), 61.

Saul, R.A., & S.H. Meredith. 2016. Beyond the Genetic Diagnosis: Providing Parents What They Want to Know. *Pediatrics in review*, *37*(7), 269–278.

Stern, A.M., N.L. Novak, N. Lira, K. O'Connor, S. Harlow, and S. Kardia. 2017. California's sterilization survivors: an estimate and call for redress. *American journal of public health*, *107*(1), 50–54.

Treff, N.R., J. Eccles, L. Lello, E. Bechor, J. Hsu, K. Plunkett et al. 2019. Utility and first clinical application of screening embryos for polygenic disease risk reduction. *Frontiers in endocrinology*, *10*, 845.

Waitzman, N.J., P.S. Romano, and R.M. Scheffler. 1994. Estimates of the economic costs of birth defects. *Inquiry*, 188–205.

Wascher, J. M., L.E. Hebert, L.R. Freedman, and D.B. Stulberg. 2018. Do women know whether their hospital is Catholic? Results from a national survey. *Contraception*, 98(6), 498–503.

Contents

Part I
Clinical Background

Chapter 1
Women, Children, Families and the Translation of Genomics in Reproductive Medicine

Ruth M. Farrell

Abstract Advances in genomic science and technology have had a significant impact on the delivery of reproductive healthcare. At the same time, these technologies generate a series of unprecedented challenges for patients and healthcare providers alike. Decision-making is at the core of the translational process bringing the use of genomics into reproductive and prenatal medicine. The full potential of these tests can only be realized if patients are able to make informed, values-based decisions about their use. This chapter examines the multi-faceted aspects that affect the translation of genomics in the reproductive context, with an emphasis on decision-making as a key component of this process, and argues that we must continue to invest in the research and development of women's decision-making around the use of these genomic technologies.

1.1 Introduction

Advances in genomic science and technology have had a significant impact on the delivery of reproductive healthcare. The newest tests can be used in the preconception, preimplantation, and prenatal stages of the reproductive healthcare spectrum to help women and families make informed decisions about their family building efforts. At the same time, these technologies generate a series of unprecedented challenges for patients and healthcare providers alike. These challenges are due, in part, to the volume and complexity of information that can be gained by their use, issues anchored in the uncertainty that comes with interpreting genomic information before birth. These challenges are also due to medical, social, and legal constructs around technology, women, children, families, and communities that impact whether and how individuals can interface with them. To complicate matters, the mode with which these technologies have traveled from the bench to the beside presents challenges of its own, a journey entrenched in the dynamics resulting from industry taking on

R. M. Farrell (✉)
Obstetrics and Gynecology, Cleveland Clinic, 9500 Euclid Avenue, OH 44195 Cleveland, USA
e-mail: farrelr@ccf.org

M. A. Allyse and M. Michie (eds.), *Born Well: Prenatal Genetics and the Future of Having Children*, The International Library of Bioethics 88,
https://doi.org/10.1007/978-3-030-82536-2_1

a lead role in how new tests are developed and implemented in the clinical arena. This chapter will examine the multi-faceted aspects that affect the translation of genomics in the reproductive context, with an emphasis on decision-making as a key component of this process.

1.2 Genetic Testing in the Reproductive Context

Genomic testing in used in the reproductive and prenatal context to identify a genomic variant that either is present in an embryo or fetus, or can be passed on to a child from one or both parents. The ultimate goal is to use the information gained from these tests to paint as accurate a picture as possible about outcomes for a child that is not yet born. In some cases, a genetic variant can be identified before efforts are undertaken to become pregnant. Such is the case with carrier screening, which can be performed on a woman and her partner to identify a disease-conferring genetic combination that can be passed to children, and, in some cases, result in disease. (American College 2017; Norton 2017) Carrier screening tests are performed for conditions that require both members of a reproductive couple to have the gene. Individuals who carry a genetic variant leading to a disease are called carriers. Most often, a carrier does not have any knowledge of having the variant, as he or she does not experience any symptoms. Yet, when two carriers have children, there is a chance that one or more of those children will be affected by the associated condition. (Grody et al. 2001; American College 2017) Ideally, carrier should be performed in the preconception period to best inform reproductive decisions before pregnancy. This timing allows couples to make decisions about how they can go about building their families knowing about the possibility of a heritable condition. There are several options available to women and their partners if both have an identified variant. (Edwards et al. 2015; Nazareth et al. 2015; Kraft et al. 2019) Some may choose the option of using assisted reproductive technologies to conceive. This process would entail undergoing preimplantation genetic testing (PGT) to determine the presence of two copies of the variant in the embryo and, if desired, selecting embryo(s) without the variant for embryo transfer. (Technology and Medicine 2008; Basille et al. 2009; Kopelman 2007) Some couples may use information about the risk of a heritable condition to have children donor gamete(s) or embryos. Additionally, there may be some who elect to approach family building using other options (e.g., adoption or foster care) or not to have children. Others may not have access to preconception carrier screening or not consider it until the pregnancy is established. In these cases, carrier screening may be performed followed by testing of the partner if a variant is identified and then then testing of the fetus if a recessive condition is suspected.

In other cases, testing cannot be performed until efforts are underway to achieve pregnancy. A prime time point is to identify a genetic variant in an embryo before transfer and implantation. This timing allows a patient and her partner to identify if an embryo(s) carries a mutation and, then using this information, decide which embryos to have transferred with the intention to have a child free of that mutation. This type of test is performed by sampling cells from an early stage embryo created through *in vitro fertilization* (IVF). Testing may then be performed to identify a monogenic, or single-gene, disease, through a process called preimplantation genetic testing-M (PGT-M, formerly referred to as PGD). (Practice Committee 2008; Basille et al. 2009) Testing may also be performed to identify the presence of a heritable or spontaneous chromosomal aneuploidy that may be associated with a common trisomy condition (e.g., Down syndrome) or may decrease the chance of implantation. This is referred to as preimplantation genetic testing-A (PGT-A, formerly referred to as PGS).

Once the pregnancy is established, patients have the option of prenatal genetic screening or diagnostic testing. (American College, 2016a) Screening can be performed in the first or second trimester of pregnancy. Women utilize prenatal genetic screens and diagnostic tests for a number of different reasons. For some, this information will be used to decide whether to end the pregnancy if a serious abnormality is identified. For others, genetic information is used to prepare for the birth of a child with a serious medical condition. Historically, conventional screening tests have identified the pregnancy's risk of a limited number of chromosomal aneuploidies, including trisomies 21, 18, and 13. Since the introduction of cell-free DNA screening (known as cfDNA, noninvasive prenatal screening/testing, or NIPS/NIPT), it has become possible to learn about the risk of a series of other genetic conditions, including sex chromosome aneuploidies, rare autosomal aneuploidies, and microdeletions associated with clinical syndromes. (Vora and O'Brien, 2014; Wapner et al. 2015; Gil et al. 2013; Gregg et al. 2016) The benefit of screening is that it provides information about the chance of a fetal genetic variant, without the risk of injury or loss of the pregnancy; however, it is associated with a significant false-positive rate. (American College, 2016b) Thus, some patients opt for diagnostic testing, which is performed either via chorionic villus sampling in the first trimester of pregnancy or via amniocentesis in the second trimester. These tests use cells from either the placenta or the amniotic fluid to identify a variant. As is the case with cfDNA screening, it is now possible to learn about a series of different variants, with the prospect of whole-exome sequencing and whole-genome sequencing generating a volume of complex information about the fetus. This information may include variants of uncertain significance and information about conditions with variable age of onset and severity.

1.3 Translating Genomics from the Bench to the Bedside

Decision-making is at the core of the translational process bringing the use of genomics into reproductive and prenatal medicine. The full potential of these tests can only be realized if patients are able to make informed, values-based decisions about their use. At the core of this process lie the concepts of autonomy and respect for persons, components of a foundation of the ethical practice of medicine (Allyse et al. 2017).

Decision-science outlines the components of the decision-making process. An informed decision is one that is made with obtaining and understanding information material to the decision and that aligns with one's values, beliefs, and goals. With respect to the informational component of decision-making, there are several different domains for patients to understand in order to make a meaningful decision about their prenatal testing choices. The first step is to understand that testing is optional and not a required part of prenatal care. If the decision is made to proceed with testing, then patients should consider what information is desired, including what condition(s) the patients want information about, and the nature of that information (e.g., risk information compared to diagnostic information). This decision also includes the trade-offs that may be made in the process (e.g. screening with the risk of a false positive versus diagnostic testing with the risk of fetal injury or loss). Finally, this decision process includes considering management options in light of the test results. This is information that should be evidence-based and provided to a patient in a way that aligns with her needs and preferences. (Dondorp et al. 2015; Rothwell et al. 2017; Kuppermann et al. 2016).

There are several challenges to ensuring that patients have the information and support needed to make informed decisions about prenatal genetic testing. Many of these complexities have existed since the development of genetic testing, which is positioned to become more complicated with advances in genomics and the introduction of whole-exome and whole-genome sequencing. (de Jong et al. 2010; Best et al. 2018; Johnston et al. 2017).

One set of challenges pertains to the complexity and uncertainty inherent in determining outcomes for a child if a genetic variant is identified as a result of testing. Most notably, patients and clinicians often times need to have some clinical insight into the expected variant phenotype in order to meaningfully interpret a genetic testing result. However, in the reproductive context, there is limited phenotypic information that can be obtained before birth. (Vora & O'Brien, 2014; Neitzel et al. 2019) In the IVF setting, embryonic morphology may confer some information about chances of implantation but does not communicate information about expected phenotype. (American Academy 2013) Prenatal genetic testing poses similar challenges. In the prenatal context, ultrasound and other imaging modalities such as MRI at least provide some information regarding anatomical considerations. Clinical databases, if they exist, may also assist in determining a more accurate picture of outcomes based upon data from children and adults with the condition. However, as a clinical exam cannot be performed until birth, outcomes cannot be more accurately described until the neonatal period. In some cases, some of the information needed to determine outcomes will not be gained until later in childhood, when the degree of the impact of a variant upon the development of the child is understood.

Further complexity and uncertainty in determining outcomes is introduced by the growing capability of genomics to identify a range of variants. This capability includes the possibility of identifying conditions with variable expression or phenotype. At the embryonic or fetal stage, it is not possible to make this determination. Additionally, while some of the identifiable conditions may manifest at birth or in childhood, others may not develop until the adult years, at a time when medical science and technology may present options to mitigate or avoid illness. In the setting of IVF, there is also uncertainty regarding the probability that the identified variant represents all of the cellular material within the embryo. Mosaicism, a condition in which some cells contain a variant while others may not, continues to add uncertainty to the decision-making process. It is also widely recognized that genomic testing reveals variants of uncertain significance (VUS) for which clinically meaningful information about outcomes are not clearly known. (Bianchi 2015; Kitzman et al. 2012) As advances in genomic technology will make it possible to identify an increasing number of variants, it will be an ongoing question of how to incorporate knowledge of chromosomal and genomic reproductive decisions. (Kraft et al. 2019; Bianchi 2012; Bianchi et al. 2012; Mattheis et al. 2008).

Individuals and couples also face other sources of complexity and uncertainty as they formulate a sense of a genetic variant's outcomes, both for a potential child with the associated medical condition and for their future family. Outcomes are not just a function of the genetic variant itself but also of the medical and social constructs around disease and disability (Michie & Allyse 2019). For instance, over the past decade a host of new interventions to support and improve the functioning of children with disease have emerged, most prominently the expansion of occupational therapy and the field of physical medicine and rehabilitation. Prior to that, there was little in the way of support for children with a serious medical condition and their families. At the same time, there has been a growing awareness of the rights and interests of those with differing abilities and advocacy groups to speak to the needs of children and their families that provide additional levels of support. Resources and changes in physical structures have emerged in schools, place of employment, and community centers so that individuals with a condition may be able to learn, growth, and thrive in their family and community (Riggan et al. 2020). All of these factors will influence outcomes and quality of life for children with a genetic condition and their families.

Notably, patients often do not have sufficient resources to navigate the complexity and uncertainty associated with decisions about genetic testing. Studies show that pregnant women continue to struggle to obtain the information and support needed to make an informed decision about their testing options. (Nazareth et al. 2015; Piechan et al. 2016; Sheinis et al. 2017; Seven et al. 2017; Smith et al. 2018) This is a multifaceted problem. First is an issue of patients' health literacy and genetic literacy. These concepts underlie the ability for individuals to acquire, understand, and operationalize information about a health condition or choice in a meaningful way. (Gates 2004; Shieh et al. 2009) Foundational concepts in genetics and genetic testing, such as chromosome, phenotype, expressivity, and positive predictive value, can present insurmountable obstacles to informed decision-making for patients because of educational levels or lack of exposure in the context of prior medical care. (Lee et al. 2019; Ormond et al. 2009) Secondly, patients must acquire a large volume of information about the capability of genetic tests. For instance, conventional prenatal serum analyte screens identify only a limited number of conditions, including trisomies 21, 18, and 13, in addition to neural tube defects. However, using tests such as cfDNA screening or chromosomal microarray, patients may learn about many different conditions with which they have no or little familiarity or for which little clinical outcome data exist. (Wapner et al. 2012).

The challenge in the clinical setting, then, is that healthcare providers must communicate such information in an effective and meaningful way. Oftentimes, there is also limited time during the appointment to do so. Furthermore, there is a shortage of genetic counselors to meet the growing volume of patients seeking information about genetic testing and, concurrently, the expansion of testing technologies to identify a greater number of variants (Dragojlovic et al. 2021). As a result of workforce limitations, patients will often receive initial counseling about their genetic testing options from a primary healthcare provider, one who may not have the extensive knowledge, time, or resources to fully address the core components of counseling (Farrell et al., 2020b). At the same time, the internet presents patients with a range of information, only a portion of which is useful. Meanwhile, direct-to-consumer marketing of genetic tests is growing, and many of these tests are directed at individuals who are considering reproductive applications (Allyse and Chandrasekharan 2015; Agarwal et al. 2013). The quality of this information is highly variable. In addition, a number of companies offer reproductive applications of genetic testing outside of current clinical guidelines, necessitating additional efforts on the part of healthcare providers to reset the knowledge base and expectation of the role of genetic tests in the reproductive setting.

These factors raise the question of how patients and families can obtain accurate and unbiased information about their testing options. Studies show that evidence-based educational resources and decision aids are an important adjunct to the education and counseling that takes place in the clinical setting (Nagle et al. 2008; Kuppermann et al. 2009). Existing resources vary with respect to content and format, ranging from interactive educational tools to novel calculators used to determine positive predictive value of a screen result. Artificial and augmented intelligence, in the form of augmented reality interfaces involving avatars and gaming interfaces, may soon offer novel ways to improve patient support in the decision-making process. These resources can help deliver information to the patient as well as initiate a process of values confirmation in which the patient considers the different values-based aspects associated with genetic testing in reproductive contexts. In addition, they can be an avenue for patients to involve their partner or family in decisions about testing—an important aspect, as decisions made about the pregnancy may have repercussions for the family as well.

Such interventions are important mechanisms to support patients as they navigate the decision-making process. However, several aspects of the decision-making process continue to pose challenges for patients and providers. For instance, there is a lack of consensus about the concept of preparation, a factor that many women and families cite as a reason to seek genetic information about a fetus (Michie & Allyse, 2020). Information is only now just emerging about how individuals and families think about the personal utility of testing Without these data, it is difficult to determine how best to support the decision-making process when thinking about outcomes (Farrell et al., 2020a). Additionally, changes in policy and law introduce a different kind of uncertainty into decisions about genetic testing. Informed decision-making entails that patients comprehend not just what a test may uncover but also what healthcare choices they have in light of that information. In the prenatal arena, this includes the option to end the pregnancy if a serious fetal condition is identified. While the option of pregnancy termination exists in the United States, changing laws and policies about abortion provision make it increasingly difficult for patients to access safe care if they make the personal and informed decision to end the pregnancy. (Rebouché and Rothenberg 2011) For some patients, the realization of barriers to achieve healthcare in light of testing results does not come until a potentially serious problem has been identified and the limitations to obtain healthcare become apparent. Thus, the decision-making process cannot take place in a vacuum but must also recognize the barriers to healthcare that materialize at the end of the genetic testing process.

At the core of the decision-making process is the issue of choice. Whether decision-support is provided in the form of a discussion in the clinical encounter or an online decision aid, the message must be conveyed that genetic testing is a choice and that patients have the option to decline testing if it is not in line with their goals, values, and beliefs. There are several challenges to effectively actualizing this concept. Current clinical guidelines recommend that all pregnant patients, regardless of age-related risk or other factor increasing risk, should be offered prenatal aneuploidy screening and diagnostic testing. (ACOG, 2016; ACOG, 2017) Such policies are established to ensure that all patients have access to prenatal testing if desired and that the decision to undergo testing lies with the patient, not with a healthcare providers' opinion about the appropriateness of testing. However, routinization of prenatal testing may, instead, erode women's autonomous decision-making. There is also the concern that the growth of genetic testing capability may present undue pressure for patients to decline testing, making it more difficult for her to express her values and preferences with respect to the use of these technologies in her reproductive healthcare. (Johnston et al. 2017; Press and Browner 1997; Lippman 1994) The risk of iatrogenic miscarriage with prenatal diagnostic testing has also been a significant decision-making tipping point for women opting out of prenatal testing. Yet, as it becomes increasingly possible to non-invasively identify a series of variants without physical risk to the pregnancy or pregnant woman, the question will remain about how to ensure patient autonomy in initiating testing and the cascade of decisions that result from that initial decision.

The difficulty, though, is that high-stakes decisions both entrenched in uncertainty and with significant implications must be made. Despite these challenges, it is imperative to develop structures to help patients and families navigate their genetic testing choices in an informed and values-based fashion. The importance of this point cannot be underestimated. The decision to utilize genetics before pregnancy is established or in the prenatal period may profoundly alter the reproductive decisions made by individuals and families. For instance, in the case of PGT-A or PGT-M, patients must decide what embryos, if any, will be selected for transfer. (Practice Committee, 2008) If the decision is made not to transfer any of the embryos, then the patient must decide the disposition of those unused embryos. She will also be faced with a myriad of different decisions, such as whether to undergo the medical and financial costs of an additional IVF cycle(s) in an attempt to have an embryo that does not carry the variant and whether to do so using either her gametes or the gametes of her partner or with donor gametes. Each decision pathway carries important consequences. In the case of prenatal genetic testing, if a serious abnormality is identified, patients must decide whether to end the pregnancy or to continue the pregnancy, and in the latter case decide whether to plan to care for a child with a serious medical condition or to consider adoption. The decisions do not end there, as information gained about heritable genetic conditions may also heavily influence future reproductive decisions. A patient who has a heritable variant identified during pregnancy may, in turn, undergo IVF for the purpose of PGT-M to identify embryos without that variant for subsequent pregnancies. In a similar fashion, a patient who is identified as a carrier may undergo prenatal genetic testing to determine whether the fetus will be affected. In this way, genomic applications are uniquely interconnected in the reproductive context, as the choices to initiate testing at one time point may carry over into other reproductive and healthcare choices. Thus, to understand the full ramifications of genomics in the reproductive context, it is critical to consider outcomes not just for the future child and family but also for the woman, who may undergo additional procedures and take on additional risks in efforts to have a healthy child and be a "good mother. (Brown et al. 1997; Marshall et al. 2007).

1.4 Conclusion

Advances in genomics present new opportunities to improve the health and wellbeing of women, children, and families. At the same time, their clinical implementation presents unique and profound challenges for individuals and families deciding whether and how to use new genomic tests in a way that aligns with their values and beliefs. Some might say countering the challenges posed by genomics is too daunting. However, we need to ensure that patients and families can make informed decisions about genomics as they plan to have a family. It is critical to continue to invest in the research and development of women's decision-making around the use of these genomic technologies.

It is also critical to move the dialogue about reproductive applications of genetic testing forward in a productive and meaningful fashion by expanding the moral arguments around genomics in reproduction. This expansion should incorporate considerations of the health and wellbeing of women. To date, much of the discussion about the use of such technologies has had greater focus on the health and wellbeing of children or the families into which they may be born. However, with such a lens, the experiences of women are lost. Yet women's experiences are a critical part of reproductive genetics. Acquiring genetic information and reacting to it entails women deciding to undergo some procedure(s) in the effort to have a "healthy" child. Those procedures may include IVF to create embryos, invasive diagnostic testing to analyze the fetal genome, obstetric interventions to optimize outcomes, or termination of pregnancy if a serious anomaly is identified. It is also important to recognize the significance of shifting decision-making about prenatal genetic testing to the earliest weeks of pregnancy. The first trimester has become a focal point for initiating genetic testing during pregnancy, with tests such as cfDNA screening and CVS leading the way. Yet, this is also the time when most spontaneously miscarriages occur, raising the question of the impact on women when the decision is made to initiate testing but then pregnancy loss is experienced. These are important experiences for women about which more data is needed to truly inform not just the public dialogue about genomics but also the conversations that patients have with their healthcare providers and families about whether and how to use genomic technologies.

References

Agarwal, A., et al. 2013. Commercial landscape of noninvasive prenatal testing in the United States. *Prenatal Diagnosis* 33: 521–531.

Allyse, M., et al. 2017. Offering prenatal screening in the age of genomic medicine: A practical guide. *Journal of Women's Health* 26: 755–761.

Allyse, M., and S. Chandrasekharan. 2015. Too much, too soon?: Commercial provision of noninvasive prenatal screening for subchromosomal abnormalities and beyond. *Genetics in Medicine* 17: 958–961.

Academy, American, and of Pediatrics Committee on Bioethics and Committee on Genetics and American College of Medical Genetics and Genomics Social, Ethical, Legal Issues Committee. 2013. Ethical and policy issues in genetic testing and screening of children. *Pediatrics* 131: 620–622.

American College of Obstetrics and Gynecologists. 2016a. Practice bulletin no. 162: Prenatal diagnostic testing for genetic disorders. *Obstetrics and Gynecology* 127: e108–e122.

American College of Obstetrics and Gynecologists. 2016b. ACOG Practice Bulletin No. 163: Screening for Fetal Aneuploidy. *Obstetrics and Gynecology* 127: e123–e137.

American College of Obstetrics and Gynecologists. 2017. Committee opinion no. 691: Carrier screening for genetic conditions. *Obstetrics and Gynecology* 129: e41–e55.

Basille, C., et al. 2009. Preimplantation genetic diagnosis: State of the art. *European Journal of Obstetrics & Gynecology and Reproductive Biology* 145: 9–13.

Best, S., et al. 2018. Promises, pitfalls and practicalities of prenatal whole exome sequencing. *Prenatal Diagnosis* 38: 10.

Bianchi, D., and S. Az. 2015. Prepare for unexpected prenatal test results. *Nature* 522(10): 29–30.

Bianchi, D.W. 2012. From prenatal genomic diagnosis to fetal personalized medicine: Progress and challenges. *Nature Medicine* 18: 1041–1051.

Bianchi, D.W., et al. 2012. Genome-wide fetal aneuploidy detection by maternal plasma DNA sequencing. *Obstetrics & Gynecology* 119: 890–901.

Brown, S., R. Small, and J. Lumley. 1997. Being a 'good mother.' *Journal of Reproductive and Infant Psychology* 15: 185–200.

de Jong, A., et al. 2010. Non-invasive prenatal testing: Ethical issues explored. *European Journal of Human Genetics* 18: 272–277.

Dondorp, W., et al. 2015. Non-invasive prenatal testing for aneuploidy and beyond: Challenges of responsible innovation in prenatal screening. *European Journal of Human Genetics* 23: 1438–1450.

Dragojlovic, N., N. Kopac, K. Borle, et al. 2021. Utilization and uptake of clinical genetics services in high-income countries: A scoping review. *Health Policy* 125: 877–887.

Edwards, J.G., et al. 2015. Expanded carrier screening in reproductive medicine—points to consider: A joint statement of the American College of Medical Genetics and Genomics, American College of Obstetricians and Gynecologists, National Society of Genetic Counselors, Perinatal Quality Foundation, and Society for Maternal-Fetal Medicine. *Obstetrics & Gynecology* 125: 653–662.

Farrell, R.M., et al. 2020. The personal utility of cfDNA screening: Pregnant patients' experiences with cfDNA screening and views on expanded cfDNA panels. *Journal of Genetic Counseling* 29: 88–96.

Farrell, R.M., et al. 2020. Making the most of the first prenatal visit: The challenge of expanding prenatal genetic testing options and limited clinical encounter time. *Prenatal Diagnosis* 40: 1265–1271.

Gates, E.A. 2004. Communicating risk in prenatal genetic testing. *Journal of Midwifery & Women's Health* 49: 220–227.

Gil, M.M., et al. 2013. Implementation of maternal blood cell-free DNA testing in early screening for aneuploidies. *Ultrasound in Obstetrics & Gynecology* 42: 34–40.

Gregg, A.R., et al. 2016. Noninvasive prenatal screening for fetal aneuploidy, 2016 update: A position statement of the American College of Medical Genetics and Genomics. *Genetics in Medicine* 18: 1056–1065.

Grody, W.W., et al. 2001. Laboratory standards and guidelines for population-based cystic fibrosis carrier screening. *Genetics in Medicine* 3: 149–154.

Johnston, J., R. Farrell, and E. Parens. 2017. Supporting women's autonomy in prenatal testing. *The New England Journal of Medicine* 377: 505.

Kitzman JO et al. 2012. Noninvasive whole-genome sequencing of a human fetus. *Sci Transl Med* 4(137): 137ra76.

Kopelman, L.M. 2007. Using the best interests standard to decide whether to test children for untreatable, late-onset genetic diseases. *The Journal of Medicine and Philosophy* 32: 375–394.

Kraft, S.A., et al. 2019. The evolving landscape of expanded carrier screening: Challenges and opportunities. *Genetics in Medicine* 21: 790–797.

Kuppermann, M., et al. 2009. Computerized prenatal genetic testing decision-assisting tool: A randomized controlled trial. *Obstetrics and Gynecology* 113: 53–63.

Kuppermann, M., et al. 2016. Preferences regarding contemporary prenatal genetic tests among women desiring testing: Implications for optimal testing strategies. *Prenatal Diagnosis* 36: 469–475.

Lee, S., et al. 2019. Pregnancy related risk perception in pregnant women, midwives & doctors: A cross-sectional survey. *BMC Pregnancy and Childbirth* 19: 1–8.

Lippman, A. 1994. The genetic construction of prenatal testing. In *Women and prenatal testing: Facing the challenges of genetic technology(p. 9)* Columbus, Ohio State University Press.

Marshall, J.L., M. Godfrey, and M.J. Renfrew. 2007. Being a 'good mother': Managing breastfeeding and merging identities. *Social Science & Medicine* 65: 2147–2159.

Mattheis, P.J., et al. 2008. Prenatal diagnosis: Beyond decisions about termination. *The Journal of Pediatrics* 153: 728.

Michie, M. 2020. Is preparation a good reason for prenatal genetic testing? Ethical and critical questions. *Birth Defects Research* 112: 332–338.

Michie, M., and M. Allyse. 2019. Gene modification therapies: Views of parents of people with Down syndrome. *Genetics in Medicine* 21: 487.

Nagle, C. et al. 2008. Use of a decision aid for prenatal testing of fetal abnormalities to improve women's informed decision making: a cluster randomised controlled trial. *BJOG: An International Journal of Obstetrics & Gynaecology* 115: 339–347.

Nazareth, S.B., G.A. Lazarin, and J.D. Goldberg. 2015. Changing trends in carrier screening for genetic disease in the United States. *Prenatal Diagnosis* 35: 931–935.

Neitzel, D., et al. 2019. Carrier screening: Should evaluating more genes be the standard of care. *Fertility and Sterility* 111: e33–e34.

Norton, M.E. 2017. Expanded carrier screening: a rational approach to screening for rare diseases. *Obstetrics and gynecology* 130: 260–261.

Ormond, K.E., et al. 2009. Information preferences of high literacy pregnant women regarding informed consent models for genetic carrier screening. *Patient Education and Counseling* 75: 244–250.

Piechan, J.L., K.A. Hines, D.L. Koller, et al. 2016. NIPT and Informed Consent: an Assessment of Patient Understanding of a Negative NIPT Result. *J Genet Couns* 25: 1127–1137.

Practice Committee of the Society for Assisted Reproductive Technology and the Practice Committee of the American Society for Reproductive Medicine. 2008. Preimplantation genetic testing: A practice committee opinion. *Fertility and Sterility* 90: S136–S143.

Press, N., and C.H. Browner. 1997. Why women say yes to prenatal diagnosis. *Social Science & Medicine* 45: 979–989.

Rebouché, R., and K. Rothenberg. 2011. Mixed messages: The intersection of prenatal genetic testing and abortion. *Howard LJ* 55: 983.

Riggan, K.A., et al. 2020. Evaluating the risks and benefits of genetic and pharmacologic interventions for Down syndrome: Views of parents. *American Journal on Intellectual and Developmental Disabilities* 125: 1–13.

Rothwell, E., et al. 2017. Experiences among women with positive prenatal expanded carrier screening results. *Journal of Genetic Counseling* 26: 690–696.

Seven, M., et al. 2017. Women's knowledge and use of prenatal screening tests. *Journal of Clinical Nursing* 26: 1869–1877.

Sheinis, M., K. Bensimon, and A. Selk. 2018. Patients' knowledge of prenatal screening for Trisomy 21. *J Genet Couns* 27: 95–103.

Shieh, C., et al. 2009. Health Literacy and Its Association with the Use of Information Sources and with Barriers to Information Seeking in Clinic-Based Pregnant Women. *Health Care for Women International* 30: 971–988.

Smith, S.K., et al. 2018. Improving women's knowledge about prenatal screening in the era of non-invasive prenatal testing for Down syndrome–development and acceptability of a low literacy decision aid. *BMC Pregnancy and Childbirth* 18: 1–14.

Vora, N.L., and B.M. O'Brien. 2014. Noninvasive prenatal testing for microdeletion syndromes and expanded trisomies: Proceed with caution. *Obstetrics & Gynecology* 123: 1097–1099.

Wapner, R.J., Babiarz, J.E., Levy, B., et al. 2015. Expanding the scope of noninvasive prenatal testing: detection of fetal microdeletion syndromes. *Am J Obstet Gynecol* 212:332.e1–9.

Wapner, R.J., D.A. Driscoll, and J.L. Simpson. 2012. Integration of microarray technology into prenatal diagnosis: Counselling issues generated during the NICHD clinical trial. *Prenatal Diagnosis* 32: 396–400.

Chapter 2
Practicing Prenatal Medicine in a Genomic Future: How the Practice of Pediatrics May (Or May Not) Change with the Introduction of Widespread Prenatal Sequencing

Volkan Okur and Wendy K. Chung

Abstract Expanded usage of next generation sequencing technologies in prenatal medicine is advancing simultaneously around the world, and diagnosis is shifting from the postnatal to the prenatal context. Practitioners caring for mother and baby have historically dichotomized their practices into prenatal and postnatal care, but the fetal genome remains unchanged and will likely be analyzed by the same genomicists across that continuum of care. This chapter addresses ways in which the future of children and pediatric medicine could be shaped by development of and access to prenatal genomic tests and the importance of educating future parents and their providers to make informed reproductive choices, especially during the current dynamic phase of genomics in which many variants identified are not definitively interpretable. Genetics and genomic technologies have been a valuable asset to prenatal diagnosis, and the role of genetic screening and diagnosis have increased significantly in the last decade. Similarly, pediatric diagnostic testing has improved significantly with the addition of genomic testing including initially chromosome microarray and then exome/genome sequencing. As methods to analyze and interpret the genome have improved on the postnatal side, the same strategies are used increasingly although with greater challenges due in part to incomplete phenotypes on the prenatal side. As reference data sets have improved to catalog normal variants and as turn-around times have shortened to meet the clinical needs of prenatal diagnosis, it is now becoming feasible to further expand genomic prenatal screening and diagnostic testing to improve the health of children. We look forward to how the future of children and pediatric medicine could be shaped by development of and access to prenatal genomic tests and the importance of educating future parents and their providers to make informed reproductive choices, especially during the current dynamic phase of

V. Okur · W. K. Chung (✉)
Department of Pediatrics, Columbia University, New York, NY, USA
e-mail: wkc@cumc.columbia.edu

W. K. Chung
Department of Medicine, Columbia University, New York, NY, USA

M. A. Allyse and M. Michie (eds.), *Born Well: Prenatal Genetics and the Future of Having Children*, The International Library of Bioethics 88,
https://doi.org/10.1007/978-3-030-82536-2_2

genomics in which many variants identified are not definitively interpretable. Hopefully, the next generation of children will be healthier and have greater access to medical care that can prevent disease with early diagnosis of health threats.

2.1 Introduction

A major focus of genetics in pediatrics has been establishing diagnoses for children for many rare, serious medical conditions, often associated with intellectual disability/neurodevelopmental disorders (ID/NDD), congenital anomalies, problems with growth, dysmorphic features, early onset and/or family history of a condition. This group of patients comprises 35%-50% (O'Malley and Hutcheon 2007; McCandless et al. 2004) of total pediatric hospitalizations and accounts for > 50% of total hospitalization costs (McCandless et al. 2004). Although initially largely evaluated by a small number of medical geneticists, genetic counselors, and genetic laboratorians, advances in genomic diagnostic technologies have significantly improved our ability to diagnose children with these disorders and are rapidly changing the practice of pediatrics. Although not yet completely automated and scalable, continued decreases in sequencing costs, decreasing turnaround times, improvements in sequencing technology to increase read length, increased data sharing and expansion of databases of disease associated alleles and reference genomes, and improved computational tools to predict the pathogenicity of variants will continue to improve genetic diagnostics and expand the clinical utility and ease of utilization by genetic professionals, other health care providers, and patients. The length of the diagnostic odyssey will continue to decrease and increasingly will traverse the boundary from the postnatal to the prenatal setting and could shape the future of the field of pediatrics. In this chapter we will review the impact of recent advances in genomic testing and look forward to what the future impact could be on children's health and society based upon decisions made about clinical implementation of genomic testing into the prenatal practice.

2.2 Drivers of Genomic Testing Implementation

The impact of genomic testing is inextricably intertwined with our ability to prevent and/or treat rare genetic disorders and although many of these conditions are not currently curable or even treatable, the ability to correctly diagnose these conditions and understand the molecular basis for the diseases along with the advances in gene editing and other genetic manipulations will drive therapeutic advances. Furthermore, as the therapeutic windows for these disorders are defined, it will become clearer what conditions should be prioritized for presymptomatic diagnosis.

We have a robust public health infrastructure with newborn screening programs (NBS) to reliably screen 50–60 disorders (largely inborn errors of metabolism that can be detected by tandem mass spectrometry) to allow for early initiation of treatment.

As additional scalable sequencing technologies including whole genome sequencing (WGS) are utilized in a small number of pilot programs to screen newborns, there is an obvious question that arises about when the optimal time is to utilize genomic testing: preconception, prenatal (invasive and non-invasive), or neonatal patients and for which populations: population wide screening or select clinical settings with higher prior probabilities of positive results such as ultrasound abnormalities or advanced parental age. Genetic testing in the prenatal setting is, however, unlike genetic testing in any other clinical context in that the decisions that are made are heavily dependent on the values of the parents, and this phase of life is often emotionally charged and can bring out latent anxiety in prospective parents.

Having information about diagnoses prior to delivery can give families and their health care providers more time to adjust to new diagnoses, plan for specialized medical care of the newborn and beyond, and make more thoughtful and informed decisions. However, without accurate information about penetrance and expressivity of these genetic conditions (many of which are relatively new and incompletely characterized), there is a danger of pregnancy terminations of fetuses that would not have been significantly impacted or would have had treatable conditions as well as altered parent/child relationships influenced by personal beliefs about genetics and the role of genes in health, cognition, and behavior.

2.3 Historical Review of Impact of Prenatal Genetic Testing

There are 3 levels of resolution used in reproductive genetic testing and 4 different sources of samples (Table 2.1). The levels of resolution are entire chromosomes, copy number variants (CNVs) within chromosomes, and nucleotide level resolution within a gene. The source of material for testing can be directly from the fetus (amniocentesis or fetal blood) or from the placenta (chorionic villus sample) and

Table 2.1 Major prenatal indications and commonly utilized tests before next generation technologies

Indication	Test
Advanced maternal age	Chromosome analysis, FISH, qPCR
Abnormal biochemical screening	Chromosome analysis, FISH, qPCR
Ultrasound abnormality	Chromosome analysis, FISH, Sequencing, qPCR, MLPA
Positive family history	Sequencing, chromosome analysis, FISH, qPCR, MLPA
Populational predisposition	Genotyping, sequencing, MLPA

Abbreviations FISH; Fluorescent In Situ Hybridization, qPCR; quantitative Polymerase Chain Reaction, MLPA; Multiplexed Ligation-dependent Probe Amplification indirectly from the fetus as cell free DNA in the maternal plasma or circulating fetal cells. Any of these biospecimens can be used for screening of genetic conditions.

Most reproductive genetic tests have been focused on high risk populations based upon maternal age, abnormal maternal serum analytes or ultrasound findings, family history, or ethnicity to inform carrier screening for certain recessive conditions (Table 2.1). Expansion of testing to unselected populations via population based screening impacts the positive predictive value of the test as the disease prevalence decreases, and the impact only clinical utility of this decreased positive predictive value must be considered with expansion of testing.

Technological innovation has consistently served as an enabler of reproductive testing. The development of Rhogam to prevent Rh-immunization led to safer amniocenteses in the 1950s and 1960s and the development of chorionic villus sampling (CVS) in 1980s (Liley 1965; Creasman et al. 1968; Williamson 1981; Brambati and Simoni 1983). Discoveries of the chromosomal origins of aneuploidies including Down, Klinefelter, and Turner syndromes (Jacobs and Strong 1959; Lejeune et al. 1959) and the association with advanced maternal age (Hook 1976) led to population based screening for these conditions using maternal serum analytes and ultrasound markers and to the diagnosis of these conditions with fetal karyotype from amniocentesis or chorionic villus sampling (Fig. 2.1). Although the risk associated with invasive fetal samples is low (1/909 (0.11%) for amniocentesis and 1/454 (0.22%) for CVS (Akolekar et al. 2015), non-invasive aneuploidy screening using high throughput sequencing or genotyping with cell free fetal DNA (cffDNA) in the maternal plasma in the first trimester with significantly higher sensitivity and specificity (Palomaki 2011; Gregg 2013; Bianchi 2014) than serum screening or ultrasound markers, was demanded by patients and rapidly adopted by obstetricians, initially for women of advanced maternal age and possibly in the near future for all pregnant women. As new methods of screening are developed, their value increases when the new tests can serve as replacements rather than additional tests adding to health care costs. However, replacing entrenched tests can be met with resistance from the established medical system. Women have been generally accepting of cffDNA to screen for aneuploidy, in part because they receive information about the fetal gender early in the pregnancy and because women believe that the test provides reassurance that their baby will be healthy (Farrell 2014), and this is one of their first duties as a good future mother. Positive cffDNA screening results still require confirmation with conventional invasive fetal testing due to false positives observed with confined placental mosaicism and technical limitations of the tests. The positive predictive value of the cffDNA screening test often varies from 50 to 90% depending on the risk status of screened population and the prevalence of the condition (Taneja 2016). Ironically, with the declining number of amniocenteses and chorionic villus samplings (Larion 2014; Srebniak et al. 2017), the procedure related complication rates for amniocentesis and CVS may increase as there will be fewer experienced providers in the years to come. With fierce competition in the market, genetic laboratories have been expanding testing beyond complete aneuploidies to some of the more common copy number variants (CNVs) (Wapner 2015), with one laboratory

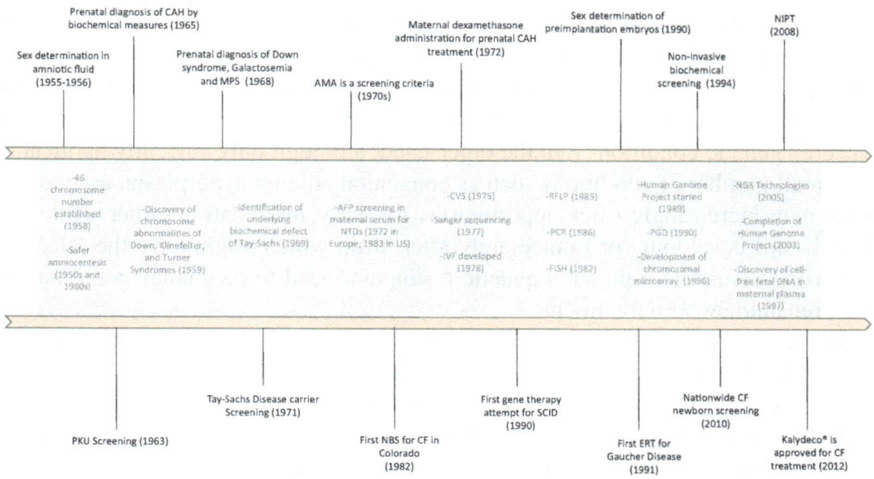

Fig. 2.1 Some important discoveries/developments in the genetic field (middle) and the prenatal breakthroughs (top) for which those discoveries/developments were utilized in prenatal diagnosis of genetic diseases in association with postnatal (bottom) diagnostic and therapeutic achievements, which altogether have served to reproductive decision making processes and initiation of effective management of genetic diseases as soon as possible. *Abbreviations* AFP: alpha-fetoprotein; AMA: Advanced maternal age; CAH: Congenital Adrenal Hyperplasia; CF: Cystic Fibrosis; CVS: Chorionic villus sampling; ERT: Enzyme replacement therapy; FISH: Fluorescent in situ hybridization IVF: in vitro fertilization; MPS: Mucopolysaccharidosis; NBS: Newborn screening; NGS: Next-generation sequencing; NTD: Neural tube defects; NIPT: Non-invasive prenatal testing; PCR: Polymerase chain reaction; PGD: Preimplantation genetic diagnosis; PKU: Phenylketonuria; RFLP: Restriction fragment length polymorphism; SCID: Severe Combined Immunodeficiency

claiming to detect all CNVs ≥ 7 Mb (Lefkowitz 2016); however, the positive predictive value for the CNV is significantly lower than aneuploidies, and should always be confirmed with a diagnostic test on chorionic villi or amniocytes (Sahoo 2016).

2.4 Effects of Next-Generation Genomic Technologies on Prenatal Diagnosis

While currently cost prohibitive to sequence the entire cell free fetal genome from a maternal sample, proof of principle pilot studies have shown that this can be done (Lo et al. 2010; Chan 2016; Kitzman et al. 2012). As the cost of sequencing declines, there will be more opportunities to expand noninvasive prenatal genetic testing for *de novo* monogenic mutations and inherited mutations, initially in high risk populations such as fetal anomalies detected on ultrasound or when parents are carriers for recessive conditions but also potentially on a large scale for fathers of advanced paternal age to detect *de novo* mutations (Goriely and Wilkie 2012). With earlier gestational age at the time of diagnosis (end of the first trimester), the bond between the woman and the fetus may not be as well developed, there may be more privacy about awareness of the pregnancy at early gestational ages and therefore less social stigma about pregnancy termination that could have the effect of greater numbers of pregnancy terminations for genetic diagnoses, potentially including less and less "severe" genetic conditions. On the other hand, although only currently applicable to a small number of conditions such as congenital adrenal hyperplasia, early diagnosis may increasingly offer opportunities for early intervention either while the fetus is still developing or immediately after birth, which might have the effect of increasing demand for prenatal genetic testing and lead to pregnancy continuation and prenatal/newborn treatment.

With the increasing availability of ultrasound to assess fetal anatomy in the second trimester, diagnostic genetic tests are valuable to determine if there is an associated genetic cause for fetuses with congenital anomalies, growth restriction, polyhydramnios, fetal hydrops, and/or soft ultrasound markers such as an echogenic focus or choroid plexus cyst. A genetic diagnosis can provide insight into prognosis, particularly for neurodevelopmental outcome, that might otherwise be difficult to predict based upon fetal anatomy alone. In addition, although a normal genetic test result reduces but never eliminates the possibility of an underlying genetic disorder, the reassurance a normal genetic result provides will influence some couples to continue a pregnancy despite a major, serious structural anomaly. For some couples making decisions about pregnancy continuation, pursuit of fetal genetic testing must proceed rapidly to provide as much information prior to the legal limit for termination which is 24 weeks in many but not all states in the US. The clinical need for comprehensive, rapid genetic testing on fetal samples led to the emergence of chromosome microarrays and now has expanded to prenatal exome/genome sequencing including a trio design with a comparison to the parental genomic information to rapidly and efficiently identify *de novo* mutations. The resolution of chromosome microarrays has improved, and some CNVs can be detected by exome/genome sequencing, such that targeted regions as small as 10 kb can be reliably identified. The diagnostic yield of prenatal chromosomal microarrays is 6–10% for all prenatal indications, with the highest diagnostic yield for ultrasound abnormalities (Wapner 2012; Callaway 2013; Oneda 2014; Lovrecic 2016).

Exome/genome sequencing have been utilized effectively in pediatrics with a minimal yield of ~ 25% of neonatal patients, and with yields approaching 50% for specific indications such as multiple congenital anomalies (Iglesias 2014; Retterer 2016). The turn-around time for pediatric exome/genome sequencing has decreased from 6 months to as little as 2 days in rare circumstances (Petrikin 2015). Applying the same genetic testing strategies of chromosome microarray and exome/genome sequencing to prenatal genetic testing could in theory approximate the yield of postnatal genetic testing for structural anomalies although generally there is less certainty about prenatal genetic diagnoses given the limits of the phenotypic data available by ultrasound. With the small series studied to date, the yield of prenatal exome/genome sequencing is 10–42% (Drury 2015; Alamillo 2015; Carss 2014; Mackie 2014). Although prenatal chromosome microarray is currently commonly covered by insurance, most prenatal exome/genome sequencing is not covered by insurance; and the cost of expedited testing is currently cost prohibitive for many patients. Increased insurance coverage for testing will almost certainly increase demand.

However, only a fraction of serious genetic conditions is associated with visible anatomic anomalies prenatally. Conditions such as intellectual disability, autism, epilepsy, muscular dystrophies, and blindness are frequently not obvious for many months or years after birth. When these conditions are a result of *de novo* mutations, screening the carrier status of the parents (see section below), will not identify fetuses at risk. Furthermore, the number of *de novo* mutations increase linearly with advancing paternal age although there is no defined threshold to determine the paternal age at which fetal exome/genome sequencing would be worthwhile in the absence of any fetal anomalies. In one large US study, the prevalence of birth defects was 1.39%, 1.47%, 1.62%, 1.68%, and 1.80% for paternal age groups of 25–34, 35–39, 40–44, 45–49, and > 50 years, respectively, and many birth defects are due to paternal *de novo* mutations (Yang 2007). Most non-familial achondroplasia patients are born to fathers who are > 35 years of age at conception (Wiener-Megnazi et al. 2012). It is even theoretically possible to screen semen samples of men of advanced paternal age prior to conception to stratify risk of having a child with a deleterious *de novo* mutation.

Addition of prenatal genomic testing must be done judiciously. As the amount of prenatal genetic information interrogated increases, the probability of identifying one or more variants of uncertain significance (VUS) increases, and it is unclear how much of this uncertain information to return to couples. *De novo* variants are more likely to be deleterious than inherited variants, especially when they are predicted to lead to loss of function and occur in genes that are dosage sensitive. However, we are still in a phase of rapid expansion of our understanding of many genes, especially genes with disruptions that lead to fetal phenotypes, and it is frequently unclear how to interpret genetic results for novel genes that have not previously been associated with human diseases. There are ongoing efforts to iteratively re-analyze variants, share data about rare variants (Boycott 2017), and perform high-throughput functional analysis of individual variants (Gasperini et al. 2016). However, there is never sufficient time in the prenatal setting to perform functional studies of novel variants and therefore there are many variants that are classified as VUS. Although VUS were routinely reported for prenatal chromosome microarrays, with the massive number of VUS that are identified in a fetal exome/genome, it is unclear which if any VUS should be returned to patients/providers and how they will use uncertain information to make decisions. There is a concern that if information is withheld from couples and the postnatal outcome is perceived to be poor and could have been partially or completely ameliorated by provision of the prenatal information, there could be liability issues for genetic providers. If the decision is made that VUS should not be returned prenatally, perhaps the genomic data should be re-evaluated postnatally with the benefit of additional phenotypic data on the newborn. What have we learned about the impact of return of VUS on parents and providers in the prenatal setting? Mothers of children in whom uncertain prenatal CNV results were returned tend to be more perseverant, vigilant, and anxious about their child's postnatal development (Werner-Lin 2017). While reassurance from providers is important to cope with these emotions, providers vary in their knowledge and understanding of these uncertain genetic results (Reiff 2012, 2013). There are differences in preferences for uncertain information among patients, and those differences should be respected (Walser 2015; Shkedi-Rafid 2016).

The number of VUS can be minimized by limiting the number of genes analyzed by evaluating a defined panel of genes rather than an exome/genome. Such a strategy has proven effective for the prenatal diagnosis of tuberous sclerosis when cardiac rhabdomyomas are observed (Northrup and Krueger 2013) or for RASopathies when there is an increased nuchal translucency (Alamillo et al. 2012; Houweling 2010). However, because we have not yet identified the majority of the genes responsible for most congenital anomalies, such a panel strategy can currently be applied to only limited number of clinical scenarios.

Furthermore, and more ethically complex is what to do with the rest of the genomic information that may not be directly related to the indication for testing but that could have health consequences, so called incidental or secondary findings. Should the same guidelines used for postnatal testing be applied to the prenatal setting? Should the recommended ACMG list of secondary findings (Kalia et al. 2016) be routinely examined in the fetus with the expectation that all the genes on this ACMG list are medically actionable in the future for the newborn and/or one of the parents? Although these secondary findings are medically actionable at some future time (although often not until adulthood), would identification of this genetic information impact decisions about continuation of the pregnancy, anxiety of the parents, and/or parenting of the child?

2.5 Carrier Screening

Based upon birth incidences of severe recessive disorders, 1–2% of couples are estimated to both be carriers of the same recessive condition (Ropers 2012), with higher percentages of couples at risk in communities with higher frequencies of consanguinity and/or higher prevalence of founder mutations. One in 3.3 individuals of Ashkenazi ancestry in New York is a carrier for one of 16 recessive disorders commonly screened (Scott 2010). Given the success of the carrier screening program for Tay-Sachs to virtually eliminate pediatric onset Tay Sachs disease in the Jewish community (Kaback et al. 1970), there has been a rapid expansion of carrier screening of other autosomal recessive severe genetic diseases across all ethnicities as laboratories such as Counsyl have increased access to testing and significantly increased the number of autosomal recessive conditions screened, well beyond ACOG or ACMG guidelines, to ~ 100 severe disorders. Depending on the clinical laboratory, mutations are assessed by genotyping or full gene sequencing. Carrier screening for both members of the couple is ideally offered and completed prior to conception so multiple reproductive options are available including avoiding a potential marriage, refraining from having a child, adoption, donor egg or donor sperm, conceiving via *in vitro* fertilization/preimplantation genetic diagnosis (IVF/PGD), conceiving naturally and utilizing prenatal diagnosis, or accepting the risk of having an affected offspring without pursuing genetic test during the pregnancy. Practically, carrier screening is often done after conception at a first trimester prenatal visit and initially only on the mother. There are several factors that can affect selection among the many reproductive options including penetrance, disease severity, treatability, cost and burden of treatment, clinical course (age of symptom onset and age at death), insurance coverage for each option, and personal/religious beliefs (Henneman 2001; Plantinga 2016). Preimplantation genetic diagnosis is often desired but rarely covered by insurance and is therefore not a viable option for many couples.

Many treatable conditions included on the newborn screening panel are also included in some carrier screening panels and can be diagnosed prenatally in the fetus to allow prospective parents the opportunity to prepare for the special needs of the newborn including identifying an appropriate hospital for delivery, identifying specialists to care for the child after birth, learning about the condition/prognosis/treatment from providers and other families, and setting aside the appropriate financial resources and/or caregiver time to provide for the medical needs of the baby. It is yet to be determined how prenatal diagnosis of these treatable conditions impacts the outcome of the baby and family, but in theory it could be significant since the clinical course can be complicated in the newborn period. Some prospective parents may decide that the lifelong burden of treatment for some conditions is too high and will elect not to have children with the condition, and couples deserve this autonomy of reproductive decision making.

As carrier screening can easily be expanded with minimal effort, a major question is which diseases should be included in these panels? Should thresholds of penetrance and/or severity be set? If so, who should judge the severity? Until recently, there was not even consensus between the ACOG and ACMG about whether spinal muscular atrophy should be included in carrier screening (Table 2.2) (Edwards 2015; Committee Opinion No 2017). Based upon experience with Tay Sachs, many prospective parents and providers currently assume that if a condition is included on the carrier screening panel, that the condition is serious and untreatable and therefore warrants serious consideration of either alternative reproductive planning or pregnancy termination. If couples are allowed to choose what will be included in their carrier screening, will they not default to "give me everything" as long as insurance covers the cost of the test? There is already confusion when relatively benign conditions such as hypoxaluria, hereditary hemochromatosis, factor V Leiden, and glucose-6-phosphate dehydrogenase deficiency are identified in the currently available carrier screening panels, and it is unclear how couples are using information about these conditions.

With the advent of expanded pan-ethnic carrier screening, data from one laboratory showed that 17% of ~ 350,000 individuals were found to be carriers for at least one of 94 conditions. It is unclear, however, what percentage of these carriers pursued partner carrier screening and pursued reproductive planning options to avoid having affected children (Haque 2016). There has been a dramatic decrease in birth incidence and/or prevalence of some but not all diseases screened prenatally (Table

Table 2.2 Recommended conditions for prenatal carrier screening by ACMG and ACOG

Population		Committee	
Disease		Before 2017	Current
Cystic fibrosis	Pan-ethnic	Both	Both
SMA	Pan-ethnic	ACMG	Both
Hemoglobinopathies	Mediterranean, Southeast Asian, African American	ACOG	ACOG
Tay-Sachs	Ashkenazi Jewish French-Canadian Cajun	Both ACOG ACOG	Both ACOG ACOG
Canavan	Ashkenazi Jewish	Both	Both
Familial Dysautonomia	Ashkenazi Jewish	Both	Both
Bloom syndrome	Ashkenazi Jewish	ACMG	Both
Fanconi anemia type C	Ashkenazi Jewish	ACMG	Both
Gaucher disease	Ashkenazi Jewish	ACMG	Both
Mucolipidosis type IV	Ashkenazi Jewish	ACMG	Both
Niemann-Pick type A	Ashkenazi Jewish	ACMG	Both
Usher syndrome type 1F and type III	Ashkenazi Jewish	Neither	ACOG
Familial Hyperinsulinism	Ashkenazi Jewish	Neither	ACOG
Glycogen storage disease type I	Ashkenazi Jewish	Neither	ACOG
Joubert syndrome	Ashkenazi Jewish	Neither	ACOG
Maple syrupe urine disease	Ashkenazi Jewish	Neither	ACOG

2.3). The incidence of Tay-Sachs disease decreased by 90% in the Ashkenazi Jewish population by 1993 (Kaback et al. 1970). In stark contrast, according to registry data from the Cystic Fibrosis Foundation, there has been a modest decrease in the incidence of cystic fibrosis since screening began in 1991 (Fig. 2.2). It is unclear whether the birth incidence for sickle cell disease and spinal muscular atrophy have changed

Table 2.3 Effects of carrier screening on disease prevalence rates

Disease	Region or Population	Birth prevalence before screening	Screening start date	Birth prevalence after screening	References
Tay-Sachs disease	Ashkenazi Jews	1/4000	1970	<1/350.000	Kaback et al. (1993)
β-thalassemia	Mediterranean	1/250	1975	1/4000	Cao et al. (1997)
Sickle-Cell Disease	Middle Eastern	2.1/100	1992	0.4/100	Al Arrayed and Al Hajeri (2012)

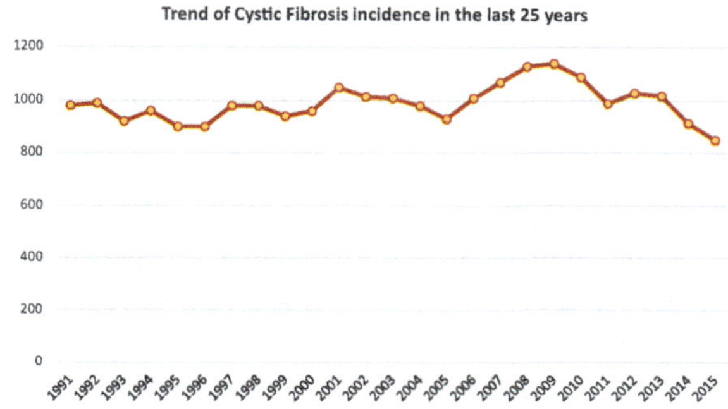

Fig. 2.2 Trend of Cystic Fibrosis (CF) incidence in the last 25 years. The approximate numbers of newly diagnosed cases were obtained from Patient Registry Annual Data Report, 2015 of Cystic Fibrosis Foundation

over time in the US. With the FDA approval of Nusinersen in 2016, an effective drug for spinal muscular atrophy when provided presymptomatically (Finkel 2016), it will be interesting to see what happens to the incidence of spinal muscular atrophy, a condition now included in the ACOG and ACMG recommended screening panel. One study suggested that universal prenatal spinal muscular atrophy carrier screening could identify 80% of SMA cases (Little 2010).

2.6 Regional and Global Differences in Contextual Factors

Expanded usage of next generation sequencing technologies in prenatal medicine is advancing simultaneously around the world; however, there are regional and global differences in disease frequency, socio-cultural, economic, religious, and political views and values that impact how reproductive genetics is implemented (Sayres 2014). In the absence of effective postnatal treatment and management options, termination of pregnancy if a genetic diagnosis is made in a fetus may be considered, but this choice depends greatly upon societal, religious, and personal beliefs. While the termination rates for trisomy 21 in the US have decreased over time, they have increased in almost all European countries and as a result the birth incidence of trisomy 21 in Europe is stable although it would have been expected to increase based on advancing age at conception of mothers in Europe (Loane 2013; Natoli 2012). There are strict laws against termination of pregnancy in some South American, African, Middle Eastern, and South Asian countries (www.worldabortionlaws.com) and as well as in some states of the US and European countries (i.e. the Republic of Ireland). If termination of a pregnancy is not an option, carrier screening works best prior to conception in a community in which preimplantation genetic diagnosis is available and accessible and/or when carrier screening is implemented prior to marriage (e.g. Dor Yeshorim in the Orthodox Jewish community). However, some genetic tests such as NIPT can only be performed once a pregnancy is conceived. Utilization of NIPT varies around the world and even within single countries is higher in patients with higher educational level, higher income, and insurance coverage (Sayres 2014; Allyse 2015). Differences in the insurance and healthcare delivery policies of different countries have significant influence on the uptake of reproductive genetic testing (Crombag 2014; Gitsels-van der Wal et al. 2014). Although they have similar national healthcare insurance systems and socio-cultural values, the uptake of prenatal Down Syndrome screening in the Netherlands is low (<30%) compared to England (74%) and Denmark (>90%), which is at least partially attributed to 'opt-in' policy in the delivery of this screening method in the Netherlands (Crombag 2014).

Availability and access to effective, acceptable treatments around the world also influences reproductive decision. In addition to trisomy 21, termination rates of Cystic Fibrosis and Gaucher disease in the US have also decreased over time in parallel to the advances in postnatal treatment and management of these conditions (Scott 2010; Natoli 2012).

2.7 Conclusion

With the expansion and improvement of preconception and prenatal genetic testing, more babies will be born well because some who would have been severely impacted will not be born and some will benefit from early treatment that will improve health. As a fetus develops and transitions to neonatal life upon delivery, there is a continuum in the care of the mother and baby that is dichotomized into prenatal and post-natal care by the practitioners providing these medical services, but the genome remains unchanged and will likely be analyzed by the same genomicists across that continuum. With the goal of providing the best quality of life to the child and the family, patient autonomy is paramount since the values and decisions of couples may vary. Preconception and prenatal genetic testing should enable improvements in outcome by allowing for more informed reproductive decision making that will likely decrease the number of births of newborns with genetic conditions as well as provide advanced diagnosis of conditions that will affect the newborn to provide the opportunity for more thoughtful planning and coordination of care by the family and the medical team that can improve outcomes in some cases. However, an under-studied consequence of learning about such diagnoses prenatally is that parents may begin to attribute the child's identity to the diagnosis and there could be self-fulfilling promises based upon parental expectations that lead to altered parenting, particularly for behavioral outcomes.

As was the case for prenatal ultrasounds providing the diagnosis of many congenital anomalies before delivery and shifting the focus of neonatologists and pediatric surgeons from diagnosis to treatment, so too will increasing prenatal genetic testing shift the focus from diagnosis to treatment and support for many rare genetic conditions. This should be a welcome advance although there could be resistance as diagnostic resources shift from postnatal to prenatal providers.

References

Akolekar, R., et al. 2015. Procedure-related risk of miscarriage following amniocentesis and chorionic villus sampling: A systematic review and meta-analysis. *Ultrasound in Obstetrics and Gynecology* 45 (1): 16–26.

Al Arrayed, S., and A. Al Hajeri. 2012. Newborn screening services in Bahrain between 1985 and 2010. *Advances in Hematology* 2012: 903219.

Alamillo, C.M., M. Fiddler, and E. Pergament. 2012. Increased nuchal translucency in the presence of normal chromosomes: What's next? *Current Opinion in Obstetrics and Gynecology* 24 (2): 102–108.

Alamillo, C.L., et al. 2015. Exome sequencing positively identified relevant alterations in more than half of cases with an indication of prenatal ultrasound anomalies. *Prenatal Diagnosis* 35 (11): 1073–1078.

Allyse, M., et al. 2015. Non-invasive prenatal testing: A review of international implementation and challenges. *Int J Womens Health* 7: 113–126.

Bianchi, D.W., et al. 2014. DNA sequencing versus standard prenatal aneuploidy screening. *New England Journal of Medicine* 370 (9): 799–808.

Boycott, K.M., et al. 2017. International Cooperation to Enable the Diagnosis of All Rare Genetic Diseases. *American Journal of Human Genetics* 100 (5): 695–705.

Brambati, B., and G. Simoni. 1983. Diagnosis of fetal trisomy 21 in first trimester. *Lancet* 1 (8324): 586.

Callaway, J.L., et al. 2013. The clinical utility of microarray technologies applied to prenatal cytogenetics in the presence of a normal conventional karyotype: A review of the literature. *Prenatal Diagnosis* 33 (12): 1119–1123.

Cao, A., Saba, L., Galanello, R., and Rosatelli, M.C. 1997. Molecular Diagnosis and Carrier Screening for beta thalassemia. *JAMA* Oct 15;278(15):1273–7.

Carss, K.J., et al. 2014. Exome sequencing improves genetic diagnosis of structural fetal abnormalities revealed by ultrasound. *Human Molecular Genetics* 23 (12): 3269–3277.

Chan, K.C., et al. 2016. Second generation noninvasive fetal genome analysis reveals de novo mutations, single-base parental inheritance, and preferred DNA ends. *Proc Natl Acad Sci U S A* 113 (50): E8159-e8168.

Committee Opinion No. 2017. 691: Carrier Screening for Genetic Conditions. *Obstetrics and Gynecology* 129 (3): e41–e55.

Creasman, W.T., R.A. Lawrence, and H.A. Thiede. 1968. Fetal complications of amniocentesis. *JAMA* 204 (11): 949–957.

Crombag, N.M., et al. 2014. Explaining variation in Down's syndrome screening uptake: Comparing the Netherlands with England and Denmark using documentary analysis and expert stakeholder interviews. *BMC Health Services Research* 14: 437.

Drury, S., et al. 2015. Exome sequencing for prenatal diagnosis of fetuses with sonographic abnormalities. *Prenatal Diagnosis* 35 (10): 1010–1017.

Edwards, J.G., et al. 2015. Expanded carrier screening in reproductive medicine-points to consider: A joint statement of the American College of Medical Genetics and Genomics, American College of Obstetricians and Gynecologists, National Society of Genetic Counselors, Perinatal Quality Foundation, and Society for Maternal-Fetal Medicine. *Obstetrics and Gynecology* 125 (3): 653–662.

Farrell, R.M., et al. 2014. It's More Than a Blood Test: Patients' Perspectives on Noninvasive Prenatal Testing. *Journal of Clinical Medicine* 3 (2): 614–631.

Finkel, R.S., et al. 2016. Treatment of infantile-onset spinal muscular atrophy with nusinersen: A phase 2, open-label, dose-escalation study. *Lancet* 388 (10063): 3017–3026.

Gasperini, M., L. Starita, and J. Shendure. 2016. The power of multiplexed functional analysis of genetic variants. *Nature Protocols* 11 (10): 1782–1787.

Gitsels-van der Wal, J.T., et al. 2014. Factors affecting the uptake of prenatal screening tests for congenital anomalies; a multicentre prospective cohort study. *BMC Pregnancy Childbirth* 14: 264.

Goriely, A., and A.O. Wilkie. 2012. Paternal age effect mutations and selfish spermatogonial selection: Causes and consequences for human disease. *American Journal of Human Genetics* 90 (2): 175–200.

Gregg, A.R., et al. 2013. ACMG statement on noninvasive prenatal screening for fetal aneuploidy. *Genetics in Medicine* 15 (5): 395–398.

Haque, I.S., et al. 2016. Modeled Fetal Risk of Genetic Diseases Identified by Expanded Carrier Screening. *JAMA* 316 (7): 734–742.

Henneman, L., et al. 2001. Participation in preconceptional carrier couple screening: Characteristics, attitudes, and knowledge of both partners. *Journal of Medical Genetics* 38 (10): 695–703.

Hook, E.B. 1976. Estimates of maternal age-specific risks of Down-syndrome birth in women aged 34–41. *Lancet* 2 (7975): 33–34.

Houweling, A.C., et al. 2010. Prenatal detection of Noonan syndrome by mutation analysis of the PTPN11 and the KRAS genes. *Prenatal Diagnosis* 30 (3): 284–286.

Iglesias, A., et al. 2014. The usefulness of whole-exome sequencing in routine clinical practice. *Genetics in Medicine* 16 (12): 922–931.

Jacobs, P.A., and J.A. Strong. 1959. A case of human intersexuality having a possible XXY sex-determining mechanism. *Nature* 183 (4657): 302–303.

Kaback, M., et al. 1993. Tay-Sachs disease--carrier screening, prenatal diagnosis, and the molecular era. An international perspective, 1970 to 1993. The International TSD Data Collection Network. *JAMA* 270(19): 2307–15.

Kalia, S.S., et al. (2017). Recommendations for reporting of secondary findings in clinical exome and genome sequencing, 2016 update (ACMG SF v2.0): a policy statement of the American College of Medical Genetics and Genomics. *Genetics Medicine* 19(2): 249–255.

Kitzman, J.O., et al. 2012. Noninvasive whole-genome sequencing of a human fetus. *Science Translational Medicine* 4(137): p. 137ra76.

Larion, S., et al. 2014. Uptake of noninvasive prenatal testing at a large academic referral center. *American Journal of Obstetrics and Gynecology* 211 (6): 651.e1–7.

Lefkowitz, R.B., et al. 2016. Clinical validation of a noninvasive prenatal test for genomewide detection of fetal copy number variants. *American Journal of Obstetrics and Gynecology* 215 (2): 227.e1-227.e16.

Lejeune, J., M. Gauthier, and R. Turpin. 1959. Human chromosomes in tissue cultures. *Comptes Rendus Hebdomadaires Des Séances De L'académie Des Sciences* 248 (4): 602–603.

Liley, A.W. 1965. AMNIOCENTESIS. *New England Journal of Medicine* 272: 731–732.

Little, S.E., et al. 2010. The cost-effectiveness of prenatal screening for spinal muscular atrophy. *American Journal of Obstetrics and Gynecology* 202 (3): 253.e1–7.

Lo, Y.M., et al. 2010. Maternal plasma DNA sequencing reveals the genome-wide genetic and mutational profile of the fetus. *Science Translational Medicine* 2(61): p. 61ra91.

Loane, M., et al. 2013. Twenty-year trends in the prevalence of Down syndrome and other trisomies in Europe: Impact of maternal age and prenatal screening. *European Journal of Human Genetics* 21 (1): 27–33.

Lovrecic, L., et al. 2016. Clinical utility of array comparative genomic hybridisation in prenatal setting. *BMC Medical Genetics* 17 (1): 81.

Mackie, F.L., et al. 2014. Exome Sequencing in Fetuses with Structural Malformations. *Journal of Clinical Medicine* 3 (3): 747–762.

McCandless, S.E., J.W. Brunger, and S.B. Cassidy. 2004. The burden of genetic disease on inpatient care in a children's hospital. *American Journal of Human Genetics* 74 (1): 121–127.

Natoli, J.L., et al. 2012. Prenatal diagnosis of Down syndrome: A systematic review of termination rates (1995–2011). *Prenatal Diagnosis* 32 (2): 142–153.

Northrup, H., and D.A. Krueger. 2013. Tuberous sclerosis complex diagnostic criteria update: Recommendations of the 2012 Iinternational Tuberous Sclerosis Complex Consensus Conference. *Pediatric Neurology* 49 (4): 243–254.

O'Malley, M., and R.G. Hutcheon. 2007. Genetic disorders and congenital malformations in pediatric long-term care. *Journal of the American Medical Directors Association* 8 (5): 332–334.

Oneda, B., et al. 2014. High-resolution chromosomal microarrays in prenatal diagnosis significantly increase diagnostic power. *Prenatal Diagnosis* 34 (6): 525–533.

Palomaki, G.E., et al. 2011. DNA sequencing of maternal plasma to detect Down syndrome: An international clinical validation study. *Genetics in Medicine* 13 (11): 913–920.

Petrikin, J.E., et al. 2015. Rapid whole genome sequencing and precision neonatology. *Seminars in Perinatology* 39 (8): 623–631.

Plantinga, M., et al. 2016. Population-based preconception carrier screening: How potential users from the general population view a test for 50 serious diseases. *European Journal of Human Genetics* 24 (10): 1417–1423.

Reiff, M., et al. 2012. What does it mean?": Uncertainties in understanding results of chromosomal microarray testing. *Genetics in Medicine* 14 (2): 250–258.

Reiff, M., et al. 2013. Physicians' perspectives on the uncertainties and implications of chromosomal microarray testing of children and families. *Clinical Genetics* 83 (1): 23–30.

Retterer, K., et al. 2016. Clinical application of whole-exome sequencing across clinical indications. *Genetics in Medicine* 18 (7): 696–704.

Ropers, H.H. 2012. On the future of genetic risk assessment. *Human Frontier Science Program* 3 (3): 229–236.

Sahoo, T., et al. 2016. Expanding noninvasive prenatal testing to include microdeletions and segmental aneuploidy: Cause for concern? *Genetics in Medicine* 18 (3): 275–276.

Sayres, L.C., et al. 2014. Demographic and experiential correlates of public attitudes towards cell-free fetal DNA screening. *Journal of Genetic Counseling* 23 (6): 957–967.

Scott, S.A., et al. 2010. Experience with carrier screening and prenatal diagnosis for 16 Ashkenazi Jewish genetic diseases. *Human Mutation* 31 (11): 1240–1250.

Shkedi-Rafid, S., et al. 2016. What results to disclose, when, and who decides? Healthcare professionals' views on prenatal chromosomal microarray analysis. *Prenatal Diagnosis* 36 (3): 252–259.

Srebniak, M.I., et al., 2017. *The influence of SNP-based chromosomal microarray and NIPT on the diagnostic yield in 10,000 fetuses with and without fetal ultrasound anomalies.* Hum Mutat, 2017.

Taneja, P.A., et al. 2016. Noninvasive prenatal testing in the general obstetric population: Clinical performance and counseling considerations in over 85 000 cases. *Prenatal Diagnosis* 36 (3): 237–243.

Walser, S.A., et al. 2015. Comparing genetic counselor's and patient's perceptions of needs in prenatal chromosomal microarray testing. *Prenatal Diagnosis* 35 (9): 870–878.

Wapner, R.J., et al. 2012. Chromosomal microarray versus karyotyping for prenatal diagnosis. *New England Journal of Medicine* 367 (23): 2175–2184.

Wapner, R.J., et al. 2015. Expanding the scope of noninvasive prenatal testing: Detection of fetal microdeletion syndromes. *American Journal of Obstetrics and Gynecology* 212 (3): 332.e1–9.

Werner-Lin, A., et al. 2017. They Can't Find Anything Wrong with Him, Yet": Mothers' experiences of parenting an infant with a prenatally diagnosed copy number variant (CNV). *American Journal of Medical Genetics. Part A* 173 (2): 444–451.

Wiener-Megnazi, Z., R. Auslender, and M. Dirnfeld. 2012. Advanced paternal age and reproductive outcome. *Asian Journal of Andrology* 14 (1): 69–76.

Williamson, R., et al. 1981. Direct gene analysis of chorionic villi: A possible technique for first-trimester antenatal diagnosis of haemoglobinopathies. *Lancet* 2 (8256): 1125–1127.

Yang, Q., et al. 2007. Paternal age and birth defects: How strong is the association? *Human Reproduction* 22 (3): 696–701.

Part II
Voices of Disability

Chapter 3
Eugenics or Not, Prenatal Genetic Testing's Common Issues Need to Be Addressed

Mark W. Leach

Abstract Critiques of prenatal genetic testing as eugenic have been debated for decades, but this strident debate can obscure ways in which persistent eugenic aspects of prenatal genetic testing can and should be addressed. Comparing arguments and professional guidelines regarding prenatal testing for genetic conditions with those regarding sex selection can provide useful insights into the ways prenatal genetic testing is offered by clinicians and administered by government programs. This chapter addresses the predominant funding models for prenatal genetic testing and ways in which these models could be improved to support broader goals of maternal and child health.

3.1 Introduction

Since its inception, prenatal genetic testing has been criticized for being eugenics. This critique is often leveled by pro-life advocates due to the high percentage of pregnancies terminated after receiving a prenatal genetic test result. Illustrating Newton's third law of motion, the pushback against this critique is made just as stridently by pro-choice advocates as well as the developers of and professionals administering prenatal genetic testing. What this chapter seeks to establish is that this heated debate should not avoid recognizing that eugenics and the current administration of prenatal genetic testing still share common issues that need to be addressed. The final section proposes how one of these issues may serve as the remedy for the common issues with eugenics.

M. W. Leach (✉)
145 Pennsylvania Ave, Louisville, KY 40206, USA
e-mail: mleach@markwleachlaw.com

M. A. Allyse and M. Michie (eds.), *Born Well: Prenatal Genetics and the Future of Having Children*, The International Library of Bioethics 88,
https://doi.org/10.1007/978-3-030-82536-2_3

3.2 The Expressivist Critique of Prenatal Genetic Testing

In their seminal work, *Prenatal Testing and Disability Rights*, Erik Parens with the Hastings Center and Professor Adrianne Asch discussed whether prenatal genetic testing was eugenics. Asch, as much a supporter of reproductive rights as she was a disability rights advocate, matter-of-factly considered abortions based on prenatal genetic testing results in "selective abortions."[1]

Eugenics means "good birth." The Eugenics Movement of the early 20th Century sought to encourage "good births" and to reduce the number of "bad births." "Bad births" were typically considered those with disabilities, to include, in the parlance of the time, feeble-mindedness. As one of the first court cases to recognize the tort of wrongful birth and wrongful life put it:

> We have alluded to the monumental implications of *Roe v. Wade,* ... one of which is the present legality of, and availability of, eugenic abortion in the proper case. Another factor of substantial proportions in "wrongful-life" litigation is the dramatic increase, in the last few decades, of the medical knowledge and skill needed to avoid genetic disaster. ... "Genetic defects represent an increasingly large part of the overall national health care burden."[2]

For most pro-life arguments, the recognition of abortions as selective against a disability and, more bluntly, as "eugenic abortions," is sufficient to condemn prenatal genetic testing. The syllogism is that most people of goodwill consider the Eugenics Movement "bad," i.e. unethical. This is why "eugenics" is a buzzword and is played like a trump card in debates about prenatal genetic testing. Therefore, if even a pro-reproductive rights academic can conclude that prenatal genetic testing results in selective abortions, then it should be settled that prenatal genetic testing is bad because eugenics is bad.

However, Asch's critique of the administration of prenatal genetic testing was not that it was wrong because it resulted in abortions. For Asch, one reason that prenatal genetic testing is ethically problematic was because it expressed a negative judgment of those with the tested-for conditions.[3] In the medical context, few associate screening or diagnostic tests with confirming something positive, e.g. "Congratulations, your test results have come back and you are destined for great height and handsomeness." Instead, the typical use of a medical test is to test for something sought to be avoided—every cancer screening is in the hopes that cancer is not detected. You test for what you don't want to have.

---

[1] Adrienne Asch, *Why I Haven't Changed My Mind about Prenatal Diagnosis: Reflections and Refinements*, in Prenatal Testing and Disability Rights (Erik Parens and Adrienne Asch ed., 2000).

[2] *Curlander v. Bio-Science Laboratories*, App., 165 Cal.Rptr. 477, 487 (1980) (*quoting Father and Mother Know Best: Defining the Liability of Physicians for Inadequate Genetic Counseling*, 87 Yale L.J. 1488, 1496 (1978). The court expressed in dicta that a disabled child could have a claim of child abuse against her parents for choosing to continue their pregnancy after prenatal diagnosis or for failing to undergo prenatal testing despite increased probability of giving birth to a child with a genetic condition.

[3] Adrianne Asch & Dorit Barlevy, Disability and Genetics: a disability critique of pre-natal testing and pre-implantation genetic diagnosis (PGD). in Encyclopedia of Life Sciences (2012).

Similarly, the expressivist critique is that by testing for certain genetic conditions, the testing expresses a negative view of those conditions as conditions to be avoided. Those screening for Down syndrome are not seeking confirmation that their pregnancy may be at a higher probability of Down syndrome; they are seeking reassurance that their pregnancy is not at a "high risk" for Down syndrome. Couple this negative association with conditions that are medically tested-for with the most common decision following a positive result being abortion and prenatal genetic testing "expresses" a negative judgment of those conditions it tests for.

The expressivist critique has its own critics. But, it should be noted that the ethics committee for the professional organization most responsible for setting the standard of care for prenatal genetic testing has recognized it as a valid concern … for one condition.

In the United States, the American College of Obstetricians & Gynecologists (ACOG) issues practice guidelines that set the standard of care, both medically and legally. ACOG's practice guidelines are readily adopted by practitioners and in turn by courts in addressing claims of medical malpractice, particularly in the case of prenatal genetic testing. In 2007, ACOG changed the standard of care for prenatal genetic testing due to the then-advance of nuchal translucency-combined screening. Before NT-combined screening, screening for aneuploidy–conditions like Down syndrome–generally was not available until the quad screen in the second trimester; NT-combined is performed in the first trimester. Prior to 2007, ACOG reserved the offer of prenatal genetic testing to mothers considered high risk, most often those mothers over the age of 35. With the advent of NT-combined, ACOG issued Practice Bulletins Nos. 77 and 88 recommending that all expectant mothers be offered prenatal genetic testing for aneuploidy.[4]

In the same year of issuing these recommendations, ACOG's ethics committee issued an opinion on sex selection.[5] The practice of selecting for sex, almost always choosing termination when a prenatal test reports "female" rather than "male", has had societal-wide impact in East Asian and Central Europe countries. Mara Hvistendahl wrote a finalist for the Pulitzer Prize, *Unnatural Selection*, detailing the imbalance in the sexes raising concern for higher rates of rapes and assaults by young men with little hope of finding a mate.[6] In response, nations like South Korea and India have instituted policies banning the use of ultrasound for diagnosing sex and gone so far as to conduct "sting" operations to identify violating practitioners. The ACOG Ethics Committee similarly came out against the use of prenatal testing for the purpose of sex selection. Its reasoning corroborates Asch's concerns about prenatal genetic testing for what are commonly-referred to as disabilities.

The ACOG Ethics Committee cited as justification for its conclusion that prenatal testing for the purpose of selecting against sex promoted sexist attitudes and was

[4] ACOG Practice Bulletin No. 77, 109 Obstet. & Gynecol. 217 (2007); ACOG Practice Bulletin No. 88, 110 Obstet. & Gynecol. 1459, 1460 (2007).

[5] ACOG Committee Opinion No. 360: Sex Selection Obstet & Gynecol 2007;109(2 Pt 1):475–8.

[6] Hvistendahl M. *Unnatural Selection: Choosing Boys Over Girls, and the Consequences of a World Full of Men.* New York: Public Affairs; 2011.

discriminatory against the sex selected against. This is the expressivist critique of prenatal genetic testing: that it promotes an able-ist attitude and is discriminatory against the conditions selected against. Therefore, this is a matter of common ground for proponents of prenatal genetic testing and its critics—they just differ over which genes or chromosomes are being selected against.

3.3 Distinctions with the Eugenics Movement

While the term "eugenic abortion" applies at the micro-level, i.e. at the patient level, generally the complaint that prenatal genetic testing is eugenics is meant to apply at the macro level. This is due to termination rates being reported ranging from a low of 61% terminating after a prenatal diagnosis (California, United States)[7] to 90 + % (France, Switzerland[8]). Headlines like the one from the Copenhagen Post that "Down Syndrome heading for extinction in Denmark"[9] further the arguments that prenatal genetic testing is eliminating those considered disabled, just like the Eugenics Movement of the early 20th Century.

Defenders of prenatal genetic testing and even academic experts on the Eugenics Movement like Paul Lombardo are quick to draw distinctions between the historical Eugenics Movement and modern-day prenatal genetic testing. Professor Lombardo wrote the book on America's Eugenics Movement, centering on the Supreme Court case of *Buck v. Bell*.[10] In that case, Carrie Buck was involuntarily sterilized under a Virginia eugenics law that permitted such violation of personal autonomy when the patient was considered "feeble-minded."

The *Buck* case provides for the distinction that modern-day prenatal genetic testing is not compulsory. Expectant women are not required to have prenatal genetic testing by professional practice guidelines or by any public laws. Instead, professional guidelines emphasize how all that is recommended is that prenatal genetic testing be offered to expectant mothers. The decision to accept or decline prenatal genetic testing should be the result of an informed choice by the patient.

This commitment to "non-directiveness" is a guiding principle for genetic counselors and medical geneticists. Genetic counselors and medical geneticists training and education emphasizes the need for assisting patients in making decisions based on their own values, rather than any biases the health care provider may have. This principle was adopted in response to the horrors committed in the name of eugenics

---

[7] Kazerouni NN, Currier B, Malm L, et al. Triple-marker prenatal screening program for chromosomal defects. Obstet Gynecol 2009;114(1):50–8.

[8] Boyd PA, Devigan C, Khoshnood B, Loane M, Garne E, Dolk H, EUROCAT Working Group. Survey of prenatal screening policies in Europe for structural malformations and chromosome anomalies, and their impact on detection and termination rates for neural tube defects and Down's syndrome. BJOG 2008;115(6):689–96.

[9] "Down Syndrome heading for extinction in Denmark," Copenhagen Post, Oct. 20, 2015.

[10] Lombardo PA. *Three Generations, No Imbeciles: Eugenics, the Supreme Court, and Buck v. Bell*. Baltimore: Johns Hopkins University Press; 2008.

as a way of assuring the public and patients that the field of genetics would not become a scientific pretext for furthering discrimination. The commitment to non-directiveness is not just a distinction with the Eugenics Movement, it was adopted as a countermeasure to eugenics.

Another distinction pointed out between the Eugenics Movement and prenatal genetic testing is the subject of each. With the Eugenics Movement, those forcibly sterilized or euthanized were living, *ex utero* human beings. The subject of prenatal genetic testing is the morally-ambiguous human fetus, which is invested with rights or none at all depending on personal and religious views and even in which state or country the pregnancy resides. Whereas involuntary surgical procedures and systematic killings is universally condemned, abortion is not just accepted, but recognized as a Constitutional right in the US and a human right in many other countries.

The final distinction defenders of prenatal genetic testing note is that, unlike the programs of the Eugenics Movement, prenatal genetic testing is not a mandated program of the state. Whereas Virginia and many other American states had laws permitting the involuntary sterilization of women and the Third Reich instituted the Holocaust as "The Final Solution," prenatal genetic testing is not mandated by law in the US or elsewhere. When women receive a prenatal test result for Down syndrome or other genetic conditions, they are not required to then have a eugenic abortion. The decision on whether to continue or terminate their pregnancy is left to them and there is no state regulation requiring one choice or the other.

3.4 Eugenic Distinctions and Modern Administration of Prenatal Genetic Testing

Defenders of prenatal genetic testing rely on the just-discussed distinctions to defend it against the eugenic complaint. Many, if not most, of those who make the eugenics complaint typically do so based just on the high termination rate, so their arguments do nothing to refute the distinctions. But how well do the distinctions hold up when examined with how prenatal genetic testing is currently administered?

A **Non-directive, autonomous choice vs. routinization, uninformed, coerced decision.**

The offering of prenatal genetic testing has not only been defended against claims of eugenics because of expectant women's autonomy, but it's been argued to be ethically obligatory because of autonomy.[11] If an expectant mother's ability to control medical decisions about her body are to be respected, then, it is argued, they must be offered the opportunity to learn whether their developing fetus has a genetic condition. And, because the decision of whether to accept prenatal genetic testing, in the first place, and whether to terminate, in the end, is the

[11] Chervenak FA, McCullough LB. Ethical considerations in first-trimester Down syndrome risk assessment. Curr Opin Obstet Gynecol 2010; 22:135–138.

expectant mother's, then prenatal genetic testing cannot be criticized for being compulsory.

These are sound arguments and would be convincing if the ideal they espouse was reflected in the reality of prenatal genetic testing's administration. However, since the dawn of prenatal genetic testing, study after study has found that women's autonomy is not respected in how prenatal genetic testing is offered. Many do not know they can decline the offer, many are unaware of what the testing is for, and many did not know they will be confronted with a decision to terminate if they follow prenatal testing to getting a diagnosis.[12] A review of these studies made the "overwhelming" conclusion that "prenatal testing does not respect a woman's autonomy."[13]

This is further reflected in the studies that counter the genetics profession's commitment to non-directiveness. A study of counselors found that while they know of the many positives that families with children with Down syndrome report and share this information in a postnatal setting, when they are counseling an expectant mother, they do not provide this information, instead focusing on medical and developmental challenges associated with the condition.[14] A study of physicians found that while some do share these positives, an even greater number emphasize the negatives about Down syndrome or outright coerce their patients to terminate their pregnancies following a prenatal diagnosis.[15]

B **Persons vs. fetuses**

The distinction of historical eugenics targeting individuals while prenatal testing deals with fetuses could be said to be a distinction without a difference from a eugenics analysis. Killing or forcibly operating on a living person is wrong, but what makes it wrong from a eugenics perspective is the reason those individuals were killed or assaulted, that reason being discrimination. Similarly, while fetuses have an ambiguous moral status and therefore abortion is permitted, what makes eugenic abortions ethically concerning is, as the ACOG Ethics Committee concluded in the case of sex selection, that they reinforce discriminatory attitudes towards those selected against.

Asch addressed this ethical distinction regarding abortion versus eugenic abortions through her concept of "any/particular." An abortion rights supporter, Asch did not have ethical concerns with "any" abortion. But what made eugenic abortions ethically problematic is that they were "particular" abortions. Women have the right to have an abortion for any or no reason. But, with eugenic abortions,

---

[12] Schoonen M, van der Zee B, Wildschut H, et al. Informing on prenatal screening for Down syndrome prior to conception. An empirical and ethical perspective. Am J Med Genet A 2012; 18A(3):485–97.

[13] Seavilleklein V. Challenging the rhetoric of choice in prenatal screening. Bioethics 2009;23:68–77.

[14] Adrienne Asch, *Disability Equality and Prenatal Testing: Contradictory or Compatible?*, 30 Fla. St. U.L. Rev. 315, 334 (2003).

[15] Dorothy C. Wertz, *Drawing Lines: Notes for Policymakers, in* Parens & Asch.

women are terminating a pregnancy because of the particular reason of selecting against a disability.[16]

The distinction between individuals and fetuses further breaks down because unlike an abortion chosen for any reason, a selective abortion is chosen because of what is expected of the life that fetus will become. The decision is not made because the fetus tested positive for Down syndrome or another genetic condition; it is made because if delivered, then that will be a child with the genetic condition.

C **State programs**

The final distinction most often made between historic eugenics and prenatal genetic testing is the lack of state involvement in the administration of prenatal genetic testing. Whereas historical eugenics involved state laws and state-actors administering eugenic programs, prenatal genetic testing is conducted like any other healthcare offering, privately between the patient and her physician. Except, there are state prenatal genetic testing programs and their justifications are identical with those of the Eugenic Movement.

The United Kingdom, Canada, Australia, and most Western European nations have a public health service which includes prenatal testing as one of the services publicly subsidized. Similarly, here in the United States, California and Iowa have state-funded prenatal genetic testing programs and Medicaid covers prenatal genetic testing in every state in the Union.[17] While patients in these nations may receive prenatal genetic testing at no or low cost to them, prenatal genetic testing is hardly free. If a mother accepts prenatal screening and then has prenatal diagnostic testing, the cost is in the thousands of dollars. Considering there are millions of women pregnant in these countries each year, these costs are significant. Add to them the cost of the abortion, which many public healthcare services subsidize, including some state Medicaid programs in the U.S., and the costs are that much higher. How are these significant publicly-subsidized costs justified? By the number of costly-lives "prevented" or "avoided."

Cost–benefit analyses are conducted for these public healthcare prenatal testing programs. Similar to other "public health" initiatives, where the cost of vaccinations are justified by the cost of treating infected patients exceeding the preventative care costs, so too are the healthcare costs of an individual with a genetic condition calculated. The millions spent on prenatal genetic testing are justified by state healthcare programs for "saving" those programs the even higher healthcare costs the analyses compute for the lifetime of an individual with the

---

[16] *See* Asch, Why I haven't changed my mind, *supra*.

[17] *See* Schoonen M, *supra*; Ranji, U., A. Salganicoff, A. M. Stewart, M. Cox, and L. Doamekpor. 2009. *The State Medicaid Coverage of Perinatal Services: Summary of State Survey Findings*. Kaiser Family Foundation. Available at: http://kaiserfamilyfoundation.files.wordpress.com/2013/01/8014.pdf.

genetic condition.[18] Researchers analyzing California's testing program have been candid in its goals and justifications:

> The California Prenatal Screening Program works to reduce the occurrence of birth defects and disability by offering prenatal screening and follow-up services to pregnant women in California.[19]

The way the program "works to reduce … birth defects and disability" with regard to genetic conditions is by identifying those conditions prenatally to allow for selective abortions.

Given this justification of preventing costly lives to offset the high costs of subsidizing prenatal genetic testing, the distinction with historical eugenics and prenatal genetic testing begins to dissolve. The Eugenics Movement's justifications for the state programs of involuntary sterilization and euthanasia was to eliminate existing or future generations of what society deemed "costly lives" or "burdens." Similarly, public healthcare subsidization of prenatal genetic testing is not premised on improving health for the mother or the fetus, but on allowing for those fetuses considered "costly" or "burdens on the system" to be eliminated.

3.5 Eugenics Concerns and Common Ground

Regardless of a person's position on prenatal genetic testing, be they critics that it facilitates eugenics or be they supporters for facilitating pregnant women's reproductive rights, it seems the distinctions the defenders make against the critics' eugenic arguments would be ones that all would support. Empowering women to make informed choices after receiving non-directive counseling are already what the professional guidelines recommend/require. But with prenatal genetic testing finishing its sixth decade, studies have yet to show this ideal being achieved. If anything, the advent of cell free DNA screening has shown that these challenges of informed providers advising patients to make informed decisions are persistent to such an extent as to be systematic and institutionalized in the health care system.

Cell-free DNA screening represented a significant change in how prenatal genetic testing was both developed and introduced to the marketplace. Whereas conventional screening and prenatal diagnostic testing had largely arisen in the field of academia and research laboratories, cfDNA screening was the product of for-profit corporations and marketed heavily. The result is that practitioners and patients alike were and are

[18] It should be noted that these cost–benefit economic analyses have their own critics for the models and estimates used. Further, these analyses fail to consider if the costs invested in prenatal genetic testing to prevent lives with genetic conditions were instead invested in the programs established to assist those individuals with more independent living, then the calculated healthcare costs would likely be much lower.

[19] Kazerouni, N. N., R. J. Currier, C. Hodgkinson, S. Goldman, F. Lorey, and M. Roberson. 2010. Ancillary benefits of prenatal maternal serum screening achieved in the California program. *Prenatal Diagnosis* 30(10): 981–987.

confused about what cfDNA screens for, how accurate it is for those conductions, and what information should accompany a test result.[20] This despite professional guidelines emphasizing how patients are to be counseled and how test results are to be delivered, and having listed resources recommended to be provided patients.[21]

When ACOG changed its recommendations following NT-combined being introduced, a study measuring compliance found that while practitioners were offering prenatal genetic testing to all patients, less than a third were offering educational materials, even though those were recommended by the same guidelines.[22] When Sequenom, the laboratory first-to-market with its cfDNA screening, launched its testing, it did so based on a study that also acknowledged that patient *and provider* information resources would be needed for patients to understand the testing and make informed choices.[23] Yet, the confusion persists and patients continue to misunderstand these tests' results.

In response, several disability support organizations and advocates around the United States introduced, lobbied for, and passed state laws requiring providing accurate information about Down syndrome and contact information for the local support organizations. When following model versions of this law, like the first one passed in Massachusetts, they are consistent with what professional guidelines require. A corresponding federal version of these laws was passed in 2008, but through compromise, was watered down to not require providing information, but authorized the Secretary for the Health and Human Services to develop materials for patients and providers. These laws, however, are almost never funded, and, in the case of the federal law, had the sole grant cut in half with nothing coming of it.[24]

The distinction with the eugenics argument yet to be addressed in this section is the role of public and private insurance subsidization and funding of prenatal genetic testing. With these policies premised and justified on explicit eugenic logic of avoiding "costly lives," the role and reasons for funding prenatal genetic testing presents the most analogous aspect to eugenics, but it may also present the opportunity to best defend against that charge.

It's a simple matter of everyday life that the cost factor influences what choices are made: whether to buy a luxury car or an affordable one; whether to rent an apartment or splurge on a large home; down to whether to by the brand name pain reliever or the generic brand. The way prenatal genetic testing has been funded has skewed this entire decision process and, perhaps if rectified, may bring the administration of

[20] Beth Daley, Oversold prenatal tests spur some to choose abortions. Boston Globe, Dec. 14, 2014.

[21] American College of Obstetricians and Gynecologists (ACOG). 2012. Noninvasive prenatal testing for fetal aneuploidy. Committee Opinion No. 545. *Obstetrics & Gynecology* 120(6): 1532–1534; Gregg, A.R., S. J. Gross, R. G. Best, et al. 2013. ACMG statement on noninvasive prenatal screening for fetal aneuploidy. *Genetics in Medicine* 15(5): 395–398.

[22] Driscoll, D.A., M. A. Morgan, J. Schulkin. 2009. Screening for Down syndrome: changing practice of obstetricians. *American Journal of Obstetrics & Gynecology*. 200(4): 459.e1—450.e9.

[23] Palomaki, G., et al., DNA sequencing of maternal plasma to detect Down syndrome: an international clinical validation study. Genet Med 2011 13(11) 913–920.

[24] Leach, MW. The Down Syndrome Information Act: Balancing the Advances of Prenatal Testing Through Public Policy. Intellect Dev Disabil 2016 Apr; 54(2); 84–93.

prenatal genetic testing closer to the ideal espoused by the professional guidelines and defenses against eugenics.

Right now, almost everywhere in the United States and in other countries with socialized medicine, what is most likely to be true is that the cost of prenatal genetic testing will be covered or subsidized. With the advances in cfDNA screening, then, the "choice" offered to an expectant mother is: would you like to have testing that is non-invasive, more accurate than ever, and at little or no cost to you? Not surprisingly, prenatal genetic testing is accepted by most expectant mothers. Then, when a positive screen is reported, they are offered diagnostic testing that is also covered or subsidized. And, if that comes back positive, in many countries, and in several states in the United States, if they choose to abort, then that, too, is covered or subsidized. Each funding decision along that chain is "justified" economically by avoiding a life deemed costlier than if the testing and abortion was not subsidized.

This argument can lead to a call for the wholesale defunding of prenatal genetic testing. If eugenics is something to be avoided and never repeated, and if the funding of prenatal genetic testing is done explicitly for eugenic reasons, then why continue the funding? Add to that the fact that the distinctions used to defend against charges of eugenics exist mainly in the ideal than in reality, with ill-informed practitioners directively counseling women who do not make informed choices, then why, again, continue to fund this? And, add to this further that there is no medical utility to prenatal genetic testing. Unlike screening for cancer which can lead to treatment or screening for some other health condition that can lead to some medical response to improve the condition, there is no prenatal genetic treatment for any condition, unless one is so crass as to view abortion as "treating" the chromosomal difference in a fetus with an aneuploidy or other genetic condition by terminating it. Given the millions and millions that are spent on funding prenatal genetic testing with no medical treatment, why continue the funding?

Such a position, however, flies in the face of most of the arguments made about prenatal genetic testing and, practically speaking, is unrealistic. Most arguments regarding funding and prenatal genetic testing instead are premised on the bioethical principle of justice to call for even more funding of it. The argument typically notes that it would be unjust for only those women who could afford prenatal genetic testing to have access to it and therefore it should be publicly subsidized to give equal access to women who otherwise would not be able to afford it. Put aside whether that money would be better invested in other prenatal care for all expectant women or even to fund the perennially underfunded state support programs for individuals with disabilities, defunding prenatal genetic testing is not likely to happen. Such a call would be shouted down as denying women their right to healthcare and it would become a political non-starter.

So, if prenatal genetic testing will continue to be publicly subsidized and if nothing changes, then prenatal genetic testing will not result in informed choices to the degree that it should and what the professional guidelines envision. If public subsidization being premised on eugenic logic is bad, then perhaps there can be a consensus that the way prenatal genetic testing is funded needs to change.

Right now, the only thing that can be counted on being funded is the testing itself—this needs to change. The funding decisions cite as their basis the ACOG professional guidelines.[25] Those same guidelines also recommend that a patient be referred to a genetic counselor when a screen result is reported for a condition.[26] Those same guidelines have identified, recommended written resources to be provided women.[27] If the public policy trends continue, soon over half of all states in the United States will have laws that require providing this same sort of information with a positive test result. If the funding is based on the recommendations of the professional guidelines, then the funding through public and private insurers should fund all the information resources that are recommended. If Medicaid and Anthem and other private insurers are going to fund NT-combined and amniocentesis, then they should fund genetic counseling and providing the written information resources about the tested-for condition. Even better, as CIGNA did with BRCA1 and BRCA2 screening: insurers should withhold funding for the testing unless the other recommended information resources of genetic counseling and written information are also provided to the patient.

3.6 Conclusion

Very likely, the argument made in this chapter will be a minority position in this collection. Those involved in prenatal genetic testing and those who support women receiving information they consider medically significant would not want to be in a system that could be argued to be fostering modern-day eugenics. Thankfully, few want to be associated with the horrors of the Eugenics Movement. And, there are many practitioners and patient experiences that can be cited as examples of how the way prenatal genetic testing was offered and accepted or declined does not qualify as eugenics. However, until funding decisions of prenatal genetic testing are not based or justified on the number of lives with Down syndrome or another tested-for condition can be eliminated and present a "savings" to the insurance or public health care system, then the charge of eugenics still applies to how prenatal genetic testing is administered. Fortunately, having identified the problem, it can also serve as the cure.

---

[25] *See e.g.* Anthem Policy #GENE.00026. 2013. Cell-free fetal DNA-based prenatal screening for aneuploidy. Available at: http://www.anthem.com/medicalpolicies/policies/mp_pw_c150729.htm.

[26] *See* ACOG PB 88 and 581, *supra.*

[27] Other American professional medical organizations have similarly issued guidelines with recommended resources. *See* Practice Guidelines for Communicating a Prenatal or Postnatal Diagnosis of Down Syndrome: Recommendations of the National Society of Genetic Counselors, J Genet Counsel (2011) 20:432–441; Gregg AR, Skotko BG, Benkendorf JL, et al. Noninvasive prenatal screening for fetal aneuploidy, 2016 update: a position statement of the American College of Medical Genetics and Genomics. Genet Med. 2016; 18:1056–1065. Regarding the latter, a follow up study found that none of the private cfDNA testing laboratories complied with all of the recommendations. *See* ·Skotko BG, Allyse MA, Leach M, Meredith S, et al. (2019) Adherence of cell-free DNA noninvasive prenatal screens to ACMG recommendations. Genet Med. 2019 Oct;21(10):2285–2292.

Instead of funding just the testing in order to prevent lives with a genetic condition, funding should be provided, and only provided, when the patient has access to proper genetic counseling and accurate, balanced, up-to-date written resources about the condition with contact information for area support organizations. If this funding change were to happen, then prenatal genetic testing could be said to not be in pursuit or based on eugenics, but instead be based on maternal and child health.

Chapter 4
The Impact of Prenatal Screening on Disability Communities and the Meaning of Disability

Louise D Bryant and Tom Shakespeare

4.1 Introduction

The advent of prenatal screening technologies has neatly paralleled the evolution of disability rights. During the 1970s and 1980s, the disability movement in many countries campaigned for barrier removal, better provision and recognition. With the adoption of the Americans with Disabilities Act 1990, the (UK) Disability Discrimination Act 1995, and cognate legislation in other countries, there finally came widespread recognition that disabled people were a discrete minority, and that society had a duty to act to ensure equal opportunities and equality. At a global level, in 2006 the UN General Assembly adopted the Convention on the Rights of Persons with Disabilities. When it came into force in 2008, the increasing number of member States who ratified it were at least in principle bound to uphold the human rights of persons with disabilities. In 2011, the World Health Organisation and World Bank issued the *World report on disability*, which provided evidence to underpin and accelerate this direction of travel.

Yet at the same time as disability was becoming seen as a social problem, not a biomedical one, and barrier removal and improved provision were slowly being put into place, the arrival of widespread prenatal screening and diagnosis arguably challenged this revisionist interpretation of disability. Rather than solving the difficulties that disabled people faced by ensuring social inclusion, prenatal interventions apparently offer a solution by removing the individuals who might have the "problem" in the first place.

L. D. Bryant
Faculty Of Medicine and Health, University of Leeds, Leeds, UK

T. Shakespeare (✉)
International Centre for Evidence in Disability, London School of Hygiene and Tropical Medicine, London, UK
e-mail: Tom.Shakespeare@lshtm.ac.uk

M. A. Allyse and M. Michie (eds.), *Born Well: Prenatal Genetics and the Future of Having Children*, The International Library of Bioethics 88,
https://doi.org/10.1007/978-3-030-82536-2_4

So the offer of serum screening for Down syndrome and spinal bifida, the development of obstetric ultrasound which can detect other fetal anomalies, the improvement of amniocentesis and chorionic villus sampling, and most recently the arrival of cell free DNA testing (otherwise known as non-invasive prenatal testing or NIPT) all increase the number of pregnancies where an increasing number of anomalies can be detected, the consequent anxiety for prospective parents, and the number of terminations of wanted pregnancies. Combining NIPT with whole genome sequencing, as is already the case in some US clinics, potentially widens the search to thousands of prenatal genetic or chromosomal anomalies, together with the developmental malformations which are often apparent on ultrasound.

No wonder prenatal screening appears to signal "eugenic elimination" to many people with disabilities and their families (Shakespeare 1999). Notwithstanding that the current prenatal services are not obviously coercive, and there appears to be no explicit government plan to eradicate disability, and it is very rare to have prominent thinkers espouse eugenic thinking (unlike in the pre-war period), there are genuine and well-founded fears of "eugenics by the back door". Some clinicians and economists have justified prenatal diagnosis and selective termination in terms of saving the costs to society of life-long support of people with disabilities. The effects of individual choice, increased screening, and both clinicians (Klein 2011) and a wider society which remains very prejudiced against disability will inevitably mean fewer births of persons with disabilities (Shakespeare 2014). As well as this practical outcome, there is a risk of disability being re-defined in terms of avoidable deficits and individual problems, rather than cultural difference and minority politics.

In other words, geneticisation (Lippman 1991) might exacerbate stigmatisation and devalue disabled people. The hurtful messages that could be conveyed by increased availability of prenatal screening—particularly if care is not taken over language, imagery and representation of disabled lives—has been summed up in the phrase "the expressivist objection": in other words, public investment in more extensive screening expresses the message that it would be better if disabled people were no longer born (Parens and Asch 2000; Klein 2011). Variations of this claim focus on the so-called "synecdoche" of viewing a disabled person not holistically, but in terms of one faulty body part or underlying genetic mutation, or on the discrimination which occurs in UK, when termination is prohibited after 24th week gestation, except in cases where the foetus is "handicapped" when the pregnancy can be terminated up until birth (Sheldon and Wilkinson 2001; McGuinness 2013). One imaginative disabled critical theorist has argued in terms of 'conserving disability' (Garland-Thomson 2012), using an implicit analogy with biodiversity, and talking about disabled people as "narrative resources" and an "experience-based counter-narrative to the modern subject's understanding of the present moment as an opportunity to shape the future". Another critic, father of a son with Down syndrome, has argued in favour of the "giftedness" of children, and the virtue of acceptance (Sandel 2007).

In ethical terms, selective termination need not always carry this burden of negative meaning. Women and men who have no intention of devaluing disabled foetuses or living disabled people come to difficult decisions, which are often driven by their circumstances: poverty, or lack of support, or worries about their other children, or simply feeling that they do not have the emotional resources to parent a child with disabilities who may require life-long support (Shakespeare 1998; Nelson 2000). If we support a woman's right to choose not to be pregnant, then, within limits, we should support her right not to continue with this particular pregnancy.

Yet at the wider societal level, the continued emphasis on genetic solutions does seem to reflect a policy injunction to promote selective termination. However, in contemporary liberal democracies, the ethos of individual choice is so powerful that it seems impossible to step back from the offer of prenatal genetic information, coupled by informed consent in the context of freely available abortion, at least until the end of the second trimester of pregnancy. Hence critics have focused on the importance of providing balanced information, and truly non-directive counselling, supporting women to test and not to test, and to terminate and not to terminate (Shakespeare 1998).

In the remainder of this chapter, we discuss empirical evidence for the attitudes of disabled people and their families to the rise of prenatal screening, before tentatively exploring whether prenatal screening will change the meaning of disability.

4.2 Attitudes of Disabled People to the Rise of Prenatal Screening

We have already highlighted the disability rights argument that widespread availability and uptake of prenatal testing expresses a negative message about the worth of disabled people and their place in society—the so-called expressivist objection (Parens and Asch 1999). This negative expression, it is said, can impact directly on the sense of self-worth of disabled individuals offending them and causing distress (Parens and Asch 2003). Despite a lack of research about the viewpoints of disabled people, some evidence for this position is available: for example, adults with Down syndrome can, understandably, find the idea of aborting babies because they have Down syndrome upsetting. It is also easy to understand that people with Down syndrome can view the widespread offer of testing to pregnant women as an expression of their being unwanted (Ward et al. 2002; Barter 2017; Barter et al. 2017).

> "Because it makes me feel like I'm not wanted in society. And no one loves us... [speaks about how her family loves her]. But the government doesn't love me, because if they did love me they wouldn't do this" and "I think it's a very sad choice that people are terminating." Sophie, woman with Down syndrome (Barter 2017). Pgs 22 & 24.

Research considering the expressivist objection within families affected by Spinal Muscular Atrophy (SMA) shows family members, including those with SMA, who consider screening are well aware of the negative message these decisions can communicate about the life-value of someone with SMA to their relatives (Boardman 2014a). It is not just about hurt feelings, though they matter (Shakespeare 2011).

The availability of prenatal screening for an ever widening range of conditions may reinforce the belief that the impairment, rather than discrimination against those with impairments, is the problem to be solved (Asch and Barlevy 2001). However, Boardman also argues that reproductive decisions are often private and hence do not necessarily communicate public messages about the acceptability of genetic conditions (Boardman 2014a).

Abortion for congenital or genetic conditions is now driven mainly by parents exercising their desire (and legal right in many countries) to avoid the birth of a child with a significant impairment (Shakespeare 2013). It can therefore be argued that the state—or private healthcare providers—are only responding to consumer demand. Yet it should be noted that many consumer demands—such as better access to fertility treatments—are not met by governments. Government financing of prenatal testing programmes, for example in the NHS, enables access to women unable to pay for private testing. Successive disability equality legislation in many countries including the UK can also be seen as evidence of a state view that disabled people are of equal value to all other citizens—once they are born. A private decision to avoid having a disabled child does not necessarily equate to a private view that disabled people are of lower value in society (Malek 2010; Murphy 2011;Shakespeare 2013). Nevertheless, individual prenatal testing and termination decisions are influenced by experiential knowledge of disability—the "characteristics of living persons with specific disabilities" (Hofmann 2017, 10). Some private decisions to terminate a pregnancy will reflect a parental view that a child with a disability/this disability is not wanted, and wantedness or otherwise is an expression of value however you look at it. Furthermore, governments do not always bow to consumer demand or deliver equitable services, for example in relation to infertility treatment or cosmetic surgery. Post-natally, screening is only offered where there is an effective intervention for the patient: prenatally, the implication is that selective termination is the right intervention, but clearly it is not good for the potential child. State decisions to finance prenatal screening programmes do therefore communicate a positive value associated with the avoidance of impairment at some level, even if this is operationalised through the enactment of individual, parental choice.

Not all disabled people see availability of prenatal testing as negative however, and in common with the non-disabled population attitudes towards prenatal testing and termination of pregnancy are diverse and complex (Boardman 2014; Gollust et al. 2003; Nuffield Council on Bioethics 2017). In a consultation about non-invasive prenatal testing with adults with Down syndrome some participants were aware that having a baby with the condition may come as a 'shock' to parents and that having a prenatal test could help them prepare. Others may feel that women have a right choose whether or not to terminate a pregnancy for Down syndrome or any other reason:

> "They are getting rid of it if they're finding out it's Down syndrome because they don't want that life for their baby or something. I mean it's a personal choice. I'm a pro-choice person. I believe what the woman wants she should get. If she doesn't wants a baby with Down's syndrome she doesn't have to… It's a woman's rights." Helen, woman with Down syndrome (Barter 2017) pg.22.

Attitudes towards prenatal testing for Spinal Muscular Atrophy (SMA) held by adults with the condition have been found to be linked to the severity of the symptoms they experience and time of symptom onset (Boardman et al. 2017). In a survey of over 80 individuals with SMA the majority were in favour of prenatal genetic screening for the condition. However, those with early onset SMA and more severe symptoms were less supportive of prenatal testing than those with late onset and milder symptoms. The group with the more severe types of SMA also viewed their experiences of disability more positively than those who had experienced life as a non-disabled person or had less significant symptoms. Individuals with relatively static impairments present from birth tend to adjust better to their condition and identify with it in comparison with those who have experienced an alternative life 'before disability' or experience periods of decline and change—being disabled is not an identity they want (Shakespeare 2006). For this group, prenatal testing is not viewed as a rejection of disabled people, rather a rejection of the negative aspects associated with impairment. This points to how a genetic condition or impairment is not always 'identity affecting', particularly if it has not been congenital (Edwards 1999).

Similarly, a study of adults with achondroplasia found that positive attitudes towards the availability of prenatal testing was associated with perceptions of a lower quality of life (Gollust et al. 2003). People with genetic conditions themselves make reproductive decisions, and some may choose to try to avoid having children sharing their genetic disability, particularly if they understand disability in terms of illness, rather than in terms of social barriers. (Boardman 2014b).

4.3 Attitudes of Families

The introduction of non-invasive prenatal genetic testing for Down syndrome into routine practice has reinvigorated the debate about the ethics of prenatal testing and renewed accusations of eugenic screening policy. Some of those most active in campaigning against the new test are those who have a child or family member with Down syndrome for example groups such as 'Don't Screen Us Out' in the UK, Downpride, and 'Saving Down syndrome' in New Zealand, Canada, France, Germany and USA. Many family members, particularly mothers of children with Down syndrome, have reacted with hurt and concern to the UK government's implementation of NIPT within the NHS, which they perceive to carry the risk of eliminating Down syndrome altogether in future. For example, 335 family members of people with Down syndrome or other trisomies responded to a Nuffield Council on Bioethics consultation on NIPT. The summary of the consultation suggested that many had had experiences or held the suspicion that:

> "some healthcare professionals don't have accurate, current understanding of what life is like for a person with Down's syndrome, should not focus overly on medical facts about the condition when discussing NIPT with women and couples, and should avoid using negative language. Balanced information should be conveyed by specially trained professionals…"

> "Some reported being asked repeatedly about screening, having refused it, being told 'scare stories' or experiencing disapproval from healthcare professionals when opting out of screening or continuing with an affected pregnancy."
>
> "Doubts expressed about the legitimacy of screening for Down's Syndrome, given nature/severity of the condition, and concerns about impact on people living with Down's Syndrome who might ultimately find themselves part of a smaller community and therefore socially isolated or excluded, may feel devalued by the existence of NIPT and the screening programme and/or may experience prejudice or discrimination." (Nuffield Council on Bioethics 2017)

As ever though, attitudes towards prenatal screening in parents and family members of disabled children and adults are diverse. Many family members support the availability of prenatal testing because they support informed reproductive choice and are aware of the challenges associated with a condition or impairment (Bryant et al. 2005; Friedman and Owen 2016; Kellogg et al. 2014). Families and individuals with a genetic condition understand that some people, maybe many people, would not choose to parent a disabled child. Some family members and individuals with a condition may themselves use testing based on their own experiences. At the same time family members and disabled people are aware that widespread availability of prenatal genetic testing communicates a message about the lower value of disabled people and makes inferences about the quality of their life and that of their families (van Schendel et al. 2017; Kellogg et al. 2014).

Having lived experience of disability, family members can find this extra knowledge increases their ambivalence about testing and the emotional burden of decision making. For parents of a child with Down syndrome considering whether or not to use screening in a future pregnancy, or the sibling of someone with a genetic condition the decision about whether or not to test is bound up with their feelings for their family member who is disabled, their personal experiences and their family context (Bryant et al. 2005; Boardman 2014; Boardman et al. 2017). Unlike those with no experience of a tested-for condition, relatives have most often (but not always) seen that families can not only cope, but thrive with a disabled child. This doesn't always mean they have no wish to avoid the situation themselves:

> It is a very complicated issue for me as I know that some genetic testing ends in terminating the pregnancy. But I am firmly pro-choice and believe that the family should have the choice to test and to take action if they feel like they need it. It's my greatest fear and I also know that I would be fine if it happened. (Friedman and Owen 2016)

Some disabled people also fear that 'blame' will become associated with having a disabled child in a society that values prenatal testing and devalues disability.

> "…My children, should they choose to have children who have an impairment, they will be viewed in a very different way. Because they will have had the choice to not do that." (Person with a genetic condition (Nuffield Council on Bioethics 2017)).

4.4 Changing Responses to Disability as a Consequence of Screening

One of the arguments against the widespread use of prenatal testing is that if fewer individuals with congenital conditions were to exist in the population, there would be less need to invest in good quality services for those who remain (Nuffield Council on Bioethics 2017). Thus it is claimed:

> "…As the number of people with disabilities decreases, it is likely that acceptance, support, and resources afforded to these people may also decrease as they (and their families, friends, and advocates) become less visible and less vocal." (Vanstone et al. 2014, p.521).

If routine use of non-invasive prenatal tests leads to a future where very few babies with Down syndrome are born, the need to meet the specific learning needs of these children might reduce, specialist skills in healthcare may well become scarcer, and related research harder to fund. While these things may not be considered a sufficient reason to restrict the reproductive choices of parents, it is important to consider if a reduction in a disabled population could lead to a lower quality of life for disabled individuals in order to take steps to mitigate this.

Evidence to support a direct link between the availability of prenatal testing with a lower quality of life for those with a tested-for condition is hard to find. On the contrary, it could be argued, that during the period in which prenatal testing has been available (in Western societies at least) there has been a greater integration of disabled people into society and improvements in public perceptions of disability (Staniland 2011). Viewed in this way there seems to be a disconnection between individual testing attitudes and behaviours and societal attitudes and behaviours towards disabled people . Alternatively, prenatal testing may not yet have had sufficient impact on the disabled population for the anticipated negative social impacts to manifest.

In the case of Down syndrome, during the same period in which prenatal screening for the condition has been introduced into routine practice maternal age has also risen steadily. As a result, with some exceptions, incidence of births of Down syndrome and other maternal age related conditions has remained relatively steady in many countries who offer screening, despite there being an increase in terminations for the condition (de Graaf et al. 2017; Kurtovic-Kozaric et al. 2016; Graaf et al. 2017; Loane et al. 2013; Maxwell et al. 2015). This may change as maternal age levels off and if non-invasive prenatal testing uptake is a as high as some anticipate (Minear et al. 2015). However, older age of both mothers and fathers are other factors which increase incidence of fetal anomaly, as is increased rate of multiple pregnancies as a result of IVF treatments, together with success in saving premature babies, who have a higher chance of being disabled. In some European countries, notably France, Spain and Switzerland high screening uptake rates have already been associated with significant reductions in the number of babies born with Down syndrome over the past 25 years (Loane et al. 2013). In countries such as Iceland and Denmark, almost all women who accept the offer of screening go on to terminate: however, a minority continue to refuse the offer of tests, and a small number of babies continue to be born in both countries. It will be important to watch what happens to Down syndrome support, service and research in these countries over the next 10 years. As they are countries with smaller populations, the impact of prenatal screening is more evident, hence fears of eliminating Down syndrome altogether.

Decisions about whether or not to use prenatal testing or selective termination cannot be separated from attitudes and beliefs about bringing up a child with that condition within the particular social context (Lawson 2006). In many low and middle income countries, social and educational support for disabled people is very limited (Chandrasekharan et al. 2014), and even in wealthy countries stigmatising attitudes are pervasive (Enea-Drapeau et al. 2012; Bryant et al. 2011). Negative stereotypes about disability, and attitudes towards disabled people are known to be associated with intentions to test for and terminate an affected pregnancy (Bryant et al. 2010; Lawson 2006; Lawson and Walls-Ingram 2010).

Research in the area of intergroup contact theory show that high quality contact with people with a disability is associated with more positive attitudes towards this group, which begins in childhood (MacMillan et al. 2014; Keith et al. 2015; Pettigrew et al. 2011). It could be proposed that over time a significant reduction in the number of disabled people would reduce opportunities for high quality interaction, which in turn is associated with more negative attitudes. However care should be taken when proposing this cause and effect conclusion—it is quality of interaction, rather than quantity that is the most important aspect and those with close relationships with disabled people hold diverse attitudes, as has already been demonstrated.

4.5 Conclusion

The meaning of disability is changing. Quality of life for people with Down syndrome has changed considerably over the last 40 years, thanks to improved support, better healthcare, more access to education and the possibilities of rewarding employment (Buckley and Buckley 2008). This translates into evidence of good outcomes for both individuals and families (Slotko et al. 2011, 2016). It would be unduly positive to view disability as a neutral difference, but no longer need it be considered to be a tragedy. Instead, it is perhaps best regarded as a predicament—something that makes life a bit more complicated, entails some losses and difficulties, but perhaps also some gains and joys (Shakespeare 2006). However, more work is required until the incomplete knowledge and outdated attitudes of some of the medical profession (Klein 2011) and many health policy-makers come up to date with contemporary realities. More research, and advocacy, is needed to capture and share the views of people living with conditions that might be preventable prenatally (Boardman et al. 2017), although it is important to note how heterogeneous these views are likely to be.

If the two approaches cannot be harmonised, then the future is one of more victim-blaming, more profits for NIPT companies, more invasive diagnosis (and associated iatrogenic miscarriage), more terminations of wanted pregnancies, and quite possibly more devaluing of disabled people and their families. This is the message of Marteau and Drake's speculative paper on "attributions for disability", (1995) where evidence was found that in cases where a mother of a disabled child was thought to have failed to screen and selective terminate, her situation was viewed with less sympathy and more blame. In a health system based on private medical insurance, the pressure on individuals to avoid disability may become stronger.

In the future, disabled children may be born into families who actively choose to avoid prenatal screening—or into families without the financial resources to afford the screening tests. In parts of East Asia where social attitudes toward intellectual disability are predominantly negative and family sizes small (Choi and Van Riper 2016), prenatal screening uptake and termination rates for Down syndrome and other chromosomal conditions are high (Allyse et al. 2015; Leung et al. 2009; Deng et al. 2015). However, currently non-invasive tests are provided only to those who can afford—or who wish to—pay for the more accurate test in these countries. If having a baby with a particularly condition becomes associated with those of lower social status, this is likely to increase the desire to use testing in those with the financial resources to avoid it. This in itself may have an impact on the future quality of life of disabled individuals.

In the world of disability much of the positive change has come about through the efforts of those with a direct personal interest—and often the personal or financial resources to make things happen (Wright and Taylor 2014; Burke et al. 2017). One reasons for improved awareness and support for children with Down syndrome, in Western countries at least, is that a disproportionate number of parents of affected children are older, have higher levels of education and are more financially secure than average (Hodapp 2007). Parents have demanded access to mainstream education and fought against outdated stereotypes of people with Down syndrome. In a parallel world where no prenatal testing exists, many more children with Down syndrome would be born into families with the means to drive for positive change; it is interesting to consider what services might look like in that scenario.

References

Allyse, M., M.A. Minear, E. Berson, S. Sridhar, M. Rote, A. Hung, and S. Chandrasekharan. 2015. Non-Invasive Prenatal Testing: A Review Of International Implementation And Challenges. *International Journal of Women's Health,* 7: 113.

Asch, A. & D. Barlevy. 2012. Disability And Genetics: A Disability Critique Of Pre-Natal Testing And Pre-Implantation Genetic Diagnosis (PGD). *ELS.* John Wiley & Sons, Ltd.

Barter, B., and R. Hastings. 2017. *Consultation With Individuals With Down Syndrome About Non Invasive Prenatal Testing (Nipt).* London: Mencap.

Barter, B., R.P. Hastings, R. Williams & J.C. Huws. 2017. Perceptions And Discourses Relating To Genetic Testing: Interviews With People With Down Syndrome. *Journal Of Applied Research In Intellectual Disabilities,* 30 (2): 395–406.

Boardman, F.K. 2014a. The Expressivist Objection To Prenatal Testing: The Experiences Of Families Living With Genetic Disease. *Social Science & Medicine,* 107: 18–25.

Boardman, F.K. 2014b. Experiential Knowledge Of Disability, Impairment And Illness: The Reproductive Decisions Of Families Genetically At Risk. *Health* 18 (5): 476–491.

Boardman, F.K., P.J. Young & F.E. Griffiths. 2018. Impairment Experiences, Identity And Attitudes Towards Genetic Screening: The Views Of People With Spinal Muscular Atrophy. *Journal Of Genetic Counseling,* 27 (1): 69–84
Bryant, L.D., S. Ahmed, M. Ahmed, H. Jafri & Y. Raashid. 2011. 'All Is Done By Allah'. Understandings Of Down Syndrome And Prenatal Testing In Pakistan. *Social Science & Medicine* 72 (8): 1393–1399.
Bryant, L.D., J.M. Green & J. Hewison. 2005. Attitudes Towards Prenatal Diagnosis And Termination In Women Who Have A Sibling With Down's Syndrome. *Journal Of Reproductive And Infant Psychology* 23 (2): 179–196.
Bryant, L.D., J.M. Green & J. Hewison. 2010. The Role Of Attitudes Towards The Targets Of Behaviour In Predicting And Informing Prenatal Testing Choices *Psychology And Health,* 25 (10): 1175–1194.
Buckley, F., and S. Buckley. 2008. Wrongful Deaths And Rightful Lives—Screening For Down Syndrome, *Down Syndrome Research And Practice* 12 (2): 79–86.
Burke, M.M., L. Sandman, B. Perez & M. O'leary. 2017. The Phenomenon Of Legislative Advocacy Among Parents Of Children With Disabilities. *Journal Of Research In Special Educational Needs.* 18 (1): 50–58
Chandrasekharan, S., M.A. Minear, A. Hung & M.A. Allyse. 2014. Noninvasive Prenatal Testing Goes Global. *Science Translational Medicine,* 6 (231): 231fs15.
Choi, H. & M. Van Riper. 2017. Adaptation In Families Of Children With Down Syndrome In East Asian Countries: An Integrative Review. *Journal Of Advanced Nursing.* 73 (8): 1792–1806.
De Graaf, G., F. Buckley, J. Dever & B.G. Skotko. 2017. Estimation Of Live Birth And Population Prevalence Of Down Syndrome In Nine Us States. *American Journal Of Medical Genetics Part A.* 173 (10): 2710–2719.
Deng, C., L. Yi, Y. Mu, J. Zhu, Y. Qin, X. Fan, Y. Wang, Q. Li & L. Dai. 2015. Recent trends in the birth prevalence of down syndrome in China: impact of prenatal diagnosis and subsequent terminations. *Prenatal Diagnosis.* 35 (4): 311–318.
Edwards, S.D. 1999. *Disability: Definitions, Value and Identity.* London, Crc Press.
Enea-Drapeau, C., M. Carlier, and P. Huguet. 2012. Tracking subtle stereotypes of children with trisomy 21: From Facial-feature-based to implicit stereotyping. *PLoS ONE* 7 (4): E34369.
Friedman, C. & A.L. Owen. 2016. Siblings Of Disabled Peoples' Attitudes Toward Prenatal Genetic Testing And Disability: A Mixed Methods Approach. *Disability Studies Quarterly,* 36 (3).
Garland-Thomson, R. 2012. The case for conserving disability. *Bioethical Inquiry,* 9: 339–355.
Gollust, S.E., R.E. Thompson, H. C. Gooding & B.B. Biesecker. 2003. Living with Achondroplasia: Attitudes toward population screening and correlation with quality of life. *Prenatal Diagnosis* 23 (12): 1003–1008.
Graaf, G., J. Engelen, A. Gijsbers, R. Hochstenbach, M. Hoffer, A. Kooper, B. Sikkema-Raddatz, M. Srebniak, A. Kevie-Kersemaekers & L. Zutven. 2017. Estimates of live birth prevalence of children with down syndrome in the period 1991–2015 In The Netherlands. *Journal Of Intellectual Disability Research,* 61 (5): 461–470.
Hodapp, R.M. 2007. Families of persons with down syndrome: New perspectives, findings, and research and service needs. *Developmental Disabilities Research Reviews* 13 (3): 279–287.
Hofmann, B. 2017. 'You Are Inferior!' Revisiting The Expressivist Argument. *Bioethics,* 31 (7): 505–514.
Keith, J.M., L. Bennetto & R.D. Rogge. 2015. The relationship between contact and attitudes: Reducing prejudice toward individuals with intellectual and developmental disabilities. *Research In Developmental Disabilities,* 47: 14–26.
Kellogg, G., L. Slattery, L. Hudgins & K. Ormond. 2014. Attitudes of mothers of children with down syndrome towards noninvasive prenatal testing. *Journal Of Genetic Counseling,* 23 (5): 805–813.
Klein, D.A. 2011. Medical disparagement of the disability experience: Empirical evidence for the expressivist objection, *AJOB Primary Research,* 2 (2): 8–20.

Kurtovic-Kozaric, A., L. Mehinovic, R. Malesevic, S. Mesanovic, T. Jaros, M. Stomornjak-Vukadin, M. Mackic-Djurovic, S. Ibrulj, I. Kurtovic-Basic and M. Kozaric. 2016. Ten-Year trends in prevalence of down syndrome in a developing country: Impact of the maternal age and prenatal screening. *European Journal Of Obstetrics & Gynecology And Reproductive Biology* 206: 79–83.

Lawson, K., and S.A. Walls-Ingram. 2010. Selective abortion for Down syndrome: The relation between the quality of intergroup contact, parenting expectations, and willingness to terminate. *Journal of Applied Social Psychology,* 40 (3): 554–578.

Lawson, K. L. 2006. Expectations of the parenting experience and willingness to consider selective termination for down syndrome *Journal Of Reproductive And Infant Psychology* 24: 43–59.

Leung, T.Y., L.W. Chan, L.W. Law, D.S. Sahota, T.Y. Fung, T.N. Leung and T.K. Lau. 2009. First trimester combined screening for Trisomy 21 In Hong Kong: Outcome Of The First 10,000 Cases. *The Journal Of Maternal-Fetal & Neonatal Medicine,* 22 (4): 300–304.

Lippman, A. 1991. Prenatal genetic testing and screening: constructing needs and reinforcing inequalities. *American Journal Of Law And Medicine* 17(1/2): 15–50.

Loane, M., J.K. Morris, M.-C. Addor, L. Arriola, J. Budd, B. Doray, E. Garne, M. Gatt, M. Haeusler, B. Khoshnood, K. Klungsoyr Melve, A. Latos-Bielenska, B. Mcdonnell, C. Mullaney, M. O'mahony, A. Queiser-Wahrendorf, J. Rankin, A. Rissmann, C. Rounding, J. Salvador, D. Tucker, D. Wellesley, L. Yevtushok & H. Dolk. 2013. Twenty-Year trends in the prevalence of down syndrome and other trisomies in Europe: Impact of maternal age and prenatal screening. *European Journal of Human Genetics,* 21 (1): 27–33.

Macmillan, M., M. Tarrant, C. Abraham and C. Morris. 2014. The Association between children's contact with people with disabilities and their attitudes towards disability: A systematic review. *Developmental Medicine & Child Neurology* 56 (6): 529–546.

Malek, J. 2010. Deciding against disability: Does the use of reproductive genetic technologies express disvalue for people with disabilities? *Journal Of Medical Ethics* 36 (4): 217–221.

Marteau, T.M., and H. Drake. 1995. Attributions for disability: The influence of genetic screening, *Social Science And Medicine* 40 (8): 1127–32.

Maxwell, S., C. Bower, and P. O'leary. 2015. Impact of prenatal screening and diagnostic testing on trends in down syndrome births and terminations in Western Australia 1980 To 2013. *Prenatal Diagnosis* 35 (13): 1324–1330.

Mcguinness, S. 2013. Law, reproduction, and disability: Fatally 'Handicapped'? *Medical Law Review* 21: 213–492.

Minear, M.A., C. Lewis, S. Pradhan, and S. Chandrasekharan. 2015. Global perspectives on clinical adoption of Nipt. *Prenatal Diagnosis,* 35 (10): 959–967.

Murphy, T.F. 2011. When choosing the traits of children is hurtful to others. *Journal Of Medical Ethics* 37 (2): 105–108.

Nuffield Council On Bioethics. 2017. *Non-Invasive Prenatal Testing: Ethical Issues.* London: Nuffield Council On Bioethics.

Parens, E. & A. Asch. 2000. The disability rights critique of prenatal genetic testing. *The Hastings Center Report,* 29 (5): S1–22.

Parens, E., and A. Asch. 2003. Disability rights critique of prenatal genetic testing: Reflections and recommendations. *Developmental Disabilities Research Reviews* 9 (1): 40–47.

Pettigrew, T.F., L.R. Tropp, U. Wagner & O. Christ. 2011. Recent Advances In intergroup contact theory. *International Journal Of Intercultural Relations* 35 (3): 271–280.

Sandel, M. 2007. *The case against perfection: Ethics in the age of Genetic Engineering.* Cambridge: Belknap Press of Harvard University.

Shakespeare, T. 1999. Losing the plot: Medical and activist discourses of contemporary genetics and disability, *Sociology Of Health And Illness* 21 (5): 669–688.

Shakespeare, T. 2014. *Disability rights and wrongs revisited.* London: Routledge.

Shakespeare, T.W. 2011. Choices, reasons and feelings: Prenatal diagnosis as disability dilemma. *Alter-European Journal Of Disability Research/Revue Européenne De Recherche Sur Le Handicap* 5 (1): 37–43.

Slotko, B.G., S.P. Levin, and R. Goldstein. 2011. Self-perceptions from people with down syndrome. *American Journal of Medical Genetics* 155: 2360–2369.

Slotko, B.G., Levin S.P., Macklin, E.A., and R.D. Goldstein. 2016. Family perspectives about down syndrome, *American Journal of Medical Genetics* Part A 170a: 930–941.

Staniland, L. 2011. *Public perceptions of disabled people: Evidence from The British Social Attitudes Survey 2009*. London: Office For Disability Issues Hm Government.

Van Schendel, R.V., A. Kater-Kuipers, E.H. Van Vliet-Lachotzki, W.J. Dondorp, M.C. Cornel, and L. Henneman. 2017. What do parents of children with Down Syndrome think about non-invasive prenatal testing (Nipt)? *Journal of Genetic Counseling* 26 (3): 522.

Vanstone, M., C. King, B. De Vrijer, and J. Nisker. 2014. Non-invasive preantal testing: Ethics and policy consequences. *Journal of Obstetrics and Gynaecology of Canada* 36 (6): 515–526.

Ward, L., J. Howarth, and J. Rodgers. 2002. Difference and choice: Exploring prenatal testing and the use of genetic information with people with learning difficulties. *British Journal Of Learning Disabilities* 30: 50–55.

Wright, A.C., & S. Taylor. 2014. Advocacy by parents of young children with special needs: Activities, processes, and perceived effectiveness. *Journal Of Social Service Research* 40 (5): 591–605.

Chapter 5
An Expressivist Disability Critique of the Expansion of Prenatal Genomics

Chris Kaposy

Abstract Prenatal genomics appears to be on an expansive trajectory toward universally-available, routine, whole-genome prenatal sequencing. But for people living with disabilities, this expansion of prenatal genomics may not be a welcome development. This chapter explores some of the objections arising from the community of people with disabilities, and articulates a defense of one particular form of objection: the claim that the expansion of prenatal genomics expresses negative messages about people with disabilities.

5.1 Introduction

An increasing variety of screening and diagnostic products are being offered to pregnant women as a result of advances in prenatal genomics. These advances have improved the accuracy of prenatal testing modalities, expanded the variety of indications for which testing is available, and made testing more patient-friendly. But for people living with disabilities, this expansion of prenatal genomics may not be a welcome development. Here I explore some of the objections arising from the community of people with disabilities, and articulate a defense of one particular form of objection—the claim that the expansion of prenatal genomics expresses negative messages about people with disabilities.

These disability-related critiques focus on two ways in which prenatal genomics has expanded. First, in less than a decade, noninvasive prenatal tests (NIPT) have been made available to pregnant women, and the number of genetic differences for which these tests can be used has steadily increased. Originally developed to test for Down syndrome, some new generation noninvasive tests also report on the presence of: trisomies 13 and 18, the sex of the fetus, sex chromosome differences, extra genetic material at the sub-chromosomal level, and genetic material that is missing at this level (Sequenom 2017). The "MaterniT GENOME" test marketed by Sequenom

C. Kaposy (✉)
Memorial University of Newfoundland, Newfoundland, Canada
e-mail: christopher.kaposy@med.mun.ca

M. A. Allyse and M. Michie (eds.), *Born Well: Prenatal Genetics and the Future of Having Children*, The International Library of Bioethics 88,
https://doi.org/10.1007/978-3-030-82536-2_5

Laboratories is an example (Sequenom 2017). The expansion of noninvasive tests appears to be on a trajectory towards prenatal whole-genome sequencing, a testing modality that would make it possible for prospective parents to have information about a fetus's complete genome (Munthe 2015).

A second aspect of the expansion of prenatal genomics is the possibility that NIPT and future technologies such as prenatal whole-genome sequencing will lead to more utilization of prenatal testing. NIPT for Down syndrome appears to be more accurate than previous screening tests, which could lead to a decrease in the number of pregnant women who are exposed to invasive diagnostic testing. Invasive tests such as amniocentesis and chorionic villus sampling carry a small risk of miscarriage. Because of the improvements of NIPT over previous screening tests, it is likely that more people will undergo prenatal testing. The use of NIPT is also likely to expand as coverage increases under public and private insurance plans, contributing to the perception that it is a routine prenatal intervention. The expanded use of NIPT could then lead to an increase in terminations of pregnancies because of fetal diagnoses of disability (Kaposy 2013, 2018; Nuffield Council on Bioethics 2017).

In addition to NIPT and whole-genome sequencing, the arguments presented in this chapter will touch on other technologies, such as preimplantation genetic diagnosis (PGD), in which the genetic material of embryos created through in vitro fertilization (IVF) are analyzed prior to implantation. Another relevant genomic technology is chromosomal microarray (CMA) which enables a high-resolution analysis of chromosomes for the purposes of detecting small additions and subtractions of chromosomal material (Nuffield Council on Bioethics 2017). CMA is often used after the extraction of samples through an invasive procedure such as amniocentesis.

Advances in genomics have also given us the gene-editing technology CRISPR-Cas9, which enables genetic alterations of one's offspring that are inherited and passed on to future descendants. Unlike NIPT, PGD, and CMA, CRISPR-Cas9 is currently considered a research tool and is not in clinical use. However the formidable power of this technology has engendered public debate about whether it ought to be used to reverse heritable genetic conditions, including genetic differences associated with disabilities (Baylis 2017b; International Summit on Human Gene Editing 2015).

For the most part, this chapter focuses on disability critiques directed at NIPT. I analyze the expansion of prenatal genomics in the form of NIPT as a social phenomenon that includes networks of actors, such as clinicians, the biotech industry, policy-makers who make funding decisions and who contribute to the development of practice guidelines, as well as prospective parents who are the consumers of these technological products. The *social phenomenon* of prenatal testing, which includes many actions and events that have contributed to the expansion of prenatal genomics, can be interpreted as conveying negative messages about people with disabilities, or so I will argue. When people with disabilities for which prenatal tests have been developed witness the social phenomenon of prenatal testing, they are justified in their interpretation that this networked series of actions and events expresses negative messages about them. In particular, the negative message that is eminently derivable from this social phenomenon is that people with disabilities ought not to have been born.

As Bjørn Hofmann has noted, this "expressivist objection" to prenatal testing is "somewhat unfashionable in the ethics literature" these days (Hofmann 2017, 1). But Hofmann himself, along with others, have begun to give expressivist arguments new attention (also Gyngell and Douglas 2016). Though my position is importantly different from Hofmann's, this chapter is meant to contribute to the re-invigoration of expressivist objections to prenatal testing, as part of the expansion of prenatal genomics.

To begin, I canvass some disability-based objections to the expansion of prenatal genomics that result from concerns about the consequences of the widespread use of these technologies. In particular I focus on the potential for prenatal testing technologies to contribute to the pathologization of disabilities, and the consequences of pathologization. From there I develop my argument in support of the expressivist objection to the expansion of prenatal genomic technologies. According to this argument, the social phenomenon of prenatal testing has unfolded against a backdrop of the medicalization of pregnancy and of disabilities, and this context of medicalization enables the social phenomenon to convey a discernable negative message about disabilities.

5.2 Concerns About Consequences

One main line of objection to the expansion of prenatal genomics derives from fears that this expansion will result in a reduction of people with the conditions for which there is testing – for example, conditions like Down syndrome, or sex-chromosome aneuploidies. The Down syndrome advocacy group "Don't Screen Us Out" gives voice to such an objection. The group describes the projected decrease in the population of people with Down syndrome in the UK due to the use of NIPT as "informal eugenics" (Don't Screen Us Out 2017). To those who share this concern, it might be offensive in itself that people like themselves, or people like their children, family members, or friends, are being systematically eliminated from the human population.

Decreasing populations of people with particular disabilities might have negative effects on those who live with such disabilities. For instance, some have voiced concern that decreased populations will result in a diminution of research funding devoted to such conditions. The Nuffield Council on Bioethics outlines how low prevalence of a condition or disease in a population corresponds to a low priority in research funding in several countries (Nuffield Council on Bioethics 2017, 57). A lack of research funding can translate into a lack of treatments or therapies for a disability, which can negatively affect health and well-being. Dr. Ségolène Aymé who chairs the rare disease Topic Advisory Group at the World Health Organization points out that for such diseases, "knowledge is scarce, the experts are few, the healthcare system is not organized for these patients, and the market is too small to be attractive when it comes to developing new therapies" (Aymé 2016).

Similarly, some fear that a reduction in the number of people with genetic conditions will result in a reduction in public provision for health and social support. Mary Casagrande, a Canadian mother of a child with Down syndrome, expresses her fear that "if the number of people with Down syndrome is dramatically reduced … the supports are not going to be there for people who have an intellectual disability because the need won't be there as much" (Grant 2018). Since funding for specific health care needs typical of people with cognitive disabilities are often tied to the prevalence of such disabilities in the population, appropriate funding might not be directed toward people with rarer conditions.

Some have expressed worry that the expansion of prenatal genomics and subsequent reduction in the populations of people with disabilities will translate into more bias against people with such disabilities, or social exclusion. For example, some people with autism fear that efforts to develop prenatal diagnostics for autism could erode progress toward their inclusion in society. The authors of the website "Learn from Autistics" discuss their fear that prenatal testing for autism will "likely lead to higher abortion rates and weaken whatever progress society has made towards autism acceptance" (2016). Reflecting on guidelines for the use of gene editing technologies such as CRISPR-Cas9, bioethicist Françoise Baylis notes that "The risks of increased discrimination (for example, racism, ableism, sexism) and stigmatization that accompany efforts to select for and against specific traits (particular characteristics and required qualities) are considerable" (Baylis 2017a). As an example, Baylis points out that members of the deaf community fear that "if they become fewer in number through overt efforts to ensure that they are not born, then they will experience increased discrimination. Manifestations of this discrimination might include renewed efforts to extinguish signed language and increased efforts at assimilation" (Baylis 2017a). There is strength in numbers, and the use of prenatal genomics may reduce the deaf population.

5.2.1 Pathologization and Unintended Consequences

In her book, *The Gene Machine*, Bonnie Rochman tells the story of Ryan Docherty (Rochman 2017). While in the prenatal stage, Ryan's mother had undergone an amniocentesis, and chromosomal microarray (CMA) analysis. The CMA revealed two variants of uncertain significance – one multi-gene duplication, and one multi-gene deletion. There is some evidence in the medical literature that an absence of one of the missing genes is associated with developmental and cognitive delays (Rochman 2017). These finding were significant enough for Ryan's parents that they were leaning towards terminating the pregnancy. However, a specialist in reproductive genetics reassured Ryan's parents that two variants were unlikely to have an effect. Ryan was born without any apparent cognitive disabilities (Rochman 2017).

This example shows that genomic technologies have the power to cast genetic differences as pathological. Without the influence of their specialist, Ryan's mother might well have opted for termination, thinking that the CMA had indicated that her fetus was genetically flawed. With only the bare genetic findings from the CMA, these concerns about the health of her potential child would be reasonable. Variants of uncertain significance, coupled with uncertain associations with disabilities, can be easily interpreted as genetic deficiencies, or as genetic risks.

Pathologization is not an abstract problem. It can have real effects, for instance, on the care that someone receives, on their well-being, or on their mortality. Consider the examples of trisomy 13 and trisomy 18. Unlike trisomy 21 (Down syndrome) these other trisomies have long been considered anomalies that are almost invariably fatal. However, in a recent editorial in *JAMA*, the neonatologist and ethicist John D. Lantos points out that over the past 30 years, survival rates for children born with trisomy 13 and 18 have been increasing (Lantos 2016). Referring to the latest population-based cohort study, "12.9% of children with trisomy 13 and 9.8% with trisomy 18 survived to 10 years" (Lantos 2016, 397). Mortality is still high, but thirty years ago "no reports indicated that these infants survived until age 1 year" (Lantos 2016, 397). According to Lantos, the lack of survival 30 years ago can be attributed to the fact that pediatricians were taught that these trisomies were fatal, and that they tended to withhold life-sustaining treatment from such children. The infants who nonetheless survived were institutionalized. Lantos argues that "predictions of lethality become self-fulfilling prophecies" (Lantos 2016, 397). More children with these genetic conditions survive nowadays because they are given neonatal intensive care, and their parents bring them home to live with their families. These are the same factors that have contributed to the massive increase in life-expectancy of people with Down syndrome over the past several decades (Wright 2011).

Trisomy 13 and 18 are markedly different from Ryan Docherty's gene variants. However, a legitimate disability critique of the expansion of prenatal genomics could focus on the possibility that similar processes of pathologization could take place with regard to subchromosomal variants of unknown significance. We are moving into an era in which technologies such as prenatal whole-genome sequencing will give us massive amounts of data about our children in utero. There is no guarantee that we will make responsible or informed decisions, as individuals or as a society, about such data. It is troubling that a technology such as CMA could identify a genetic difference and contribute to the (mis)interpretation of this difference as a pathology. In the case of gene variants such as Ryan's, it is unlikely that the "self-fulfilling prophecy" would be fatal. However the potentially negative consequences of pathologization cannot be clearly foreseen for all genetic differences.

5.3 Expressing a Message: Claims and Examples

The disability-based critiques I have articulated thus far focus on potential negative consequences for people with disabilities of the expansion of prenatal genomics. There is a further powerful critique of these technologies that focuses on the messages that their widespread use conveys to people with disabilities. This critique is often referred to as the "expressivist" objection. The use of these technologies is thought to express negative messages about disabilities because the technologies are often used to avoid the birth of people with disabilities.

The expressivist objection has various formulations. One version is that the use of these prenatal interventions "is an expression of disvalue for existing people" with the disabilities that are the target of testing (Hofmann 2017, p.1). Susan Wendell claims that the message sent by the widespread use of prenatal testing and selective abortion for disabilities is that "we do not want any more like you" (Wendell 1996, 153). Marsha Saxton argues that, "The message at the heart of widespread selective abortion on the basis of prenatal diagnosis is the greatest insult: some of us are 'too flawed' in our very DNA to exist; we are unworthy of being born" ([1998] 2010, 131).

Different formulations of the objection identify different individuals or groups as the purveyors of these messages. Some suggest that these harmful messages about disabilities are conveyed by the actions of individual prospective parents who choose prenatal testing or selective termination. Other formulations suggest that the messages arise from social trends (i.e. Saxton's reference to "widespread selective abortion"). The various formulations also differ slightly in the content of the message being sent. Some claim the message is about the desires of prospective parents (i.e. Wendell's interpretation: "we do not want any more like you") and others suggest that the message is about people with disabilities (i.e. Saxton's interpretation: "unworthy of being born"). The different formulations of the expressivist objection, however, share in common the claims that (1) the actions associated with testing for and selectively aborting fetuses with disabling conditions can send a message (or messages), or express a meaning, and (2) that the messages sent by these actions are negative or derogatory about people with the conditions for which people undergo testing.

In the following sections I draw upon Down syndrome as an example of a condition about which negative messages may be expressed through the social phenomenon of prenatal testing. I use this example because it is the most familiar to me, and because there has been a long history of prenatal testing and selective abortion for Down syndrome. Many of the arguments could apply equally well for other genetic conditions that correlate with cognitive disabilities, or physical disabilities, for which there are prenatal tests, or for which prenatal tests will likely be developed in the future. For example, Cri-du-chat syndrome and Wolf-Hirschhorn syndrome are conditions resulting from genetic microdeletions for which noninvasive screening tests have recently been developed (Dundorp et al. 2015). Autism is a condition with causes that are at least partly genetic, for which prenatal tests will likely be developed in the future. Though I often refer to Down syndrome, the expressivist argument I present could also apply to these conditions if prenatal testing results in high rates of selective abortion for these conditions.

Sex chromosome aneuploidies are an interesting further example. Noninvasive prenatal tests have newly become available for these conditions, such as Turner syndrome, Klinefelter syndrome (XXY) and triple-X syndrome. These aneuploidies have a variable phenotype that has been described as "generally mild" (Dundorp et al. 2015, 1443). For example, people with XYY syndrome (males with an extra Y chromosome) tend to have no physical differences compared to XY males other than a taller stature, and tend to have normal intelligence (Goobie and Prasad 2012). Some people with XYY syndrome have learning difficulties and behavioural problems, though it is difficult to assess the prevalence of these problems because cases of XYY syndrome prior to the availability of noninvasive screening typically went undetected (Goobie and Prasad 2012). Sex chromosome aneuploidies have a lower selective termination rate than Down syndrome (Boyd et al. 2011). If the selective termination rate for these conditions increases as a result of the routinization of NIPT, there would be grounds for advancing the expressivist argument, and for worrying about the likelihood that prenatal tests have pathologized these genetic differences.

5.3.1 "Official" Messages

One of the main problems to be confronted by those advancing the expressivist objection is the difficulty with attributing determinate messages to actions—such as the action of undergoing a selective termination. I will return to this issue below. However, the expressivist objection can also be directed at actual statements made by individuals, institutions, or governmental bodies. In these circumstances, there is less difficulty with raising the expressivist objection. In the UK for example, statements in the *Human Fertilisation and Embryology Act* (1990, amended 2008) and its supporting documentation make preimplantation genetic diagnosis (PGD) available only to determine whether a "serious genetic condition" is present in the embryo.[1] The Human Fertilisation and Embryology Authority keeps a list of conditions that qualify under this legislative standard of being a "serious genetic condition" (Human Fertilisation and Embryology Authority 2018). Controversially, Down syndrome is one example of such a condition (Krahn 2011). In effect, the official government position of the UK is that Down syndrome is a serious genetic condition. Timothy Krahn notes that.

> the HFEA licensing of PGD for Down's syndrome according to the standards established by the HFE Act 1990 (as amended 2008), sends the message that this is a "serious condition" that carries with it a significant risk of imposing significant suffering (or other compromising features) for quality of life for the affected, prospective offspring and the families of these affected offspring (Krahn 2011, 189).

Because of these messages, prospective parents would commonly be left with the impression that they should avoid bringing a child with this condition into the world.

Similarly, one of the original explanatory notes to the Bill that eventually became the *Human Fertilisation and Embryology Act* of 2008 stated that a goal of the Act was to prevent the selection of embryos that would result in a deaf child (Porter and Smith 2013). Through this explanatory note, the UK government expressed the view that prospective parents should avoid giving birth to a deaf child. The *Act* would eventually make it illegal to use IVF to do this. Christian Munthe similarly argues that publicly-funded and publicly-organized prenatal mass-screening programs that

[1] See: Human Fertilisation and Embryology Authority 2008.

designate certain disabling conditions as the targets of screening send "an implied official message that certain types of people are undesirable" (Munthe 2015).

5.3.2 Statements Made by Professionals

The expressivist objection can also be directed unproblematically at statements made by individuals. Consider some examples uncovered by the historian of medicine Ilana Löwy. Löwy has traced out the history of prenatal diagnosis in the latter part of the twentieth century. She documents how Down syndrome emerged in the medical literature as a "public health problem" that could be addressed through screening programs and selective abortion (Löwy 2014, 290). Many professionals who advanced these initiatives during this period made stigmatizing statements about Down syndrome. In 1971, epidemiologists Zena Stein and Mervin Susser characterized people with Down syndrome as living in a "state of permanent dependence that imposes a severe burden on their families and on existing forms of social organization" (Stein and Susser 1971, 650). These authors make this claim in support of a plan to systematically screen for Down syndrome. In 1973, Stein and Susser, along with Andrea Guterman considered the practical difficulties of instituting a universal screening program for Down syndrome, including the difficulty of cost. They argued that, "The lifelong care of severely retarded persons is so burdensome in almost every human dimension that no preventive program is likely to overweight the burden" (Stein, Susser, and Guterman 1973, 308). Löwy also quotes an article from 1991 that states "the prevalence of Down syndrome has major resource implications" (Sheldon and Simpson 1991, 302). Similarly, an economic study of the incidence of congenital disabilities from 1994 discusses "birth defects' economic burden to society" (Waitzman, Romano, and Scheffler 1994, 188).

More recently, an economic analysis of enabling all pregnant women in the US to have access to NIPT mentions that "trisomy 21 is the most common fetal aneuploidy and has a high survival rate, leading to high medical costs" (Benn et al. 2015). According to the authors, "decreasing termination rates was associated with a reduction in NIPT value" (Benn et al. 2015), so the economic benefit to society of NIPT is contingent upon pregnant women choosing selective termination when given a prenatal diagnosis of trisomy 21. The message being conveyed by such statements is that people with Down syndrome are a burden on their families, and on society. This explicit message, coupled with the push to screen for Down syndrome, clearly implies that such people should not be born.

Furthermore, some medical professionals continue to promote prenatal testing and selective abortion for Down syndrome in ways that express negative attitudes about people with this condition. Social science research reveals that some clinicians insist that pregnant women terminate pregnancies if given a Down syndrome diagnosis, and some perpetuate negative stereotypes about Down syndrome (for example Nelson Goff et al. 2013). These instances are direct and clear statements of disvalue about people with Down syndrome.

5.3.3 *The Message Received by People with Disabilities*

Many people with disabilities and their advocates voice the sorts of concerns about the social phenomenon of prenatal testing that are articulated by expressivist objection. A report by the Nuffield Council on Bioethics on the implementation of NIPT in the UK quotes a person with Down syndrome as stating that the use of prenatal screening for his condition "makes me feel like I'm not wanted in society and no one loves us" (Nuffield Council on Bioethics 2017, 59). The Nuffield Council interviewed various stakeholders for their report. Other respondents with genetic conditions and advocates for people living with disabilities articulated similar objections (see Sect. 2.65–2.69).

The Canadian Down Syndrome Society's VATTA self-advocacy group has created a video, "What Prenatal Testing Means to Me" (Canadian Down Syndrome Society 2014). In the video, one of the self-advocates cites the high rates of selective termination for Down syndrome, and pointedly asks, "has anyone ever wondered how that makes us feel?". The question answers itself. Similarly, the "Don't Screen Us Out" advocacy group in the UK has clearly interpreted the widespread use of prenatal testing for Down syndrome as an effort to eliminate people with this condition through "screening" them out. The message they are receiving is that people with Down syndrome should not exist (Don't Screen Us Out 2017).

5.4 The Social Phenomenon of Prenatal Testing

Many different actors are involved in prenatal testing and selective abortion. Aside from the prospective parents who make testing and termination decisions, primary care physicians, obstetricians, midwives, and genetic counsellors take part in these activities. These professionals are also involved in developing guidelines about the use of prenatal genomic technologies, along with other actors such as epidemiologists, public health officials, ethicists, and managers of health care organizations. As we have seen, guidelines and policies are a particularly sensitive form of communication subject to the expressivist objection. In addition to these groups, scientists and industry executives are involved in developing and marketing new prenatal tests, some of which can currently detect conditions that were previously undetectable prenatally. Health insurance industry executives, health systems bureaucrats, and political decision-makers are involved in determining whether the new tests will be funded through private and public health insurance plans. The motives, goals, and social forces to which each of these actors are subject can be examined through the lens of the expressivist objection. One can ask, for instance, whether a corporate decision to create a product that makes it easier to test for Down syndrome conveys any negative messages about this condition, or whether a political decision to provide public funding for such a test conveys these messages.

The fact that there can be many targets of the expressivist objection beyond the individual choices of individual prospective parents suggests that we should examine prenatal testing and selective abortion as a social phenomenon that is larger than individual choices. What I am calling the "social phenomenon" of prenatal testing encompasses many events, decisions, actions, policies: pieces of information related to prenatal testing from which one can possibly take away an underlying social message about disability.

Within the network that is subject to the expressivist objection we must include the actions of prenatal test development companies who invest large sums of money in the creation and marketing of new prenatal tests, enticed by the promise of large profits. Through these extensive efforts to develop new and more user-friendly tests these companies act on the assumption that many people value being able to identify disabilities prenatally, and that the public will use their products. We must also include the decisions of professional physician groups who develop practice guidelines for new prenatal tests. These guidelines follow a typical logic in which a restricted group of pregnant women are first deemed eligible for testing because they are considered at greater "risk" (i.e. women over 35 years of age), and then as time passes eligibility is broadened to include all pregnant women (e.g. Summers et al. 2007). The social phenomenon of prenatal testing must include as well the high rates of selective termination for certain indications—67% choose termination after being given a prenatal diagnosis of Down syndrome, according to one study, 90% according to another study (Natoli et al.2012; Mansfield et al. 1999). Another aspect of this social phenomenon is the typical routinization of prenatal testing in which women are offered prenatal tests, or these tests are administered, despite a lack of appropriate informed consent (Seavilleklein 2009; Thomas 2017). The attitude that such tests are "routine" is prevalent even though there is no prenatal treatment for the disabilities in question except termination of pregnancy, and even though the prospective parents who engage in prenatal testing in order to prepare for the possible birth of a child with a disability are a small minority. These facts suggest that clinicians who have made prenatal testing routine assume or even expect that pregnant women will terminate when they are given a prenatal diagnosis of a disability. My use of the concept of the "social phenomenon of prenatal testing" is meant to signify all of these events, decisions, policies, experiences, and actions.

5.5 Meaning and Medicalization

Since I am taking aim at a social phenomenon rather than any given individual actions, the challenge is to show that a multi-faceted group of events and choices has a more-or-less determinate meaning. I must show how a social phenomenon can mean something.

The underlying theory of meaning I will draw upon here is the Wittgenstinian theory presented by Jamie Lindemann Nelson in the article, "The Meaning of the Act: Reflections on the Expressive Force of Reproductive Decision Making and Policies" (Nelson 1998). According to Nelson, "the meaning of a symbol is a matter of how it is used, its role in a publicly shareable system of symbols" (Nelson 1998, 178).

This view is one of the hallmarks of a Wittgenstinian theory of meaning. Meaning is determined by use in a language or system of symbols. Practices such as speech acts, gestures, or actions can convey meaning by participating in a game-like activity that is guided by rules. These ideas about the rules that regulate the meaning of a practice are captured by Wittgenstein's term "language-game" (Wittgenstein [1953] 1997). The meaning of an action is determined by the role it plays as set out by the rules of a language-game. This view contrasts with theories of meaning that locate the meaning of linguistic acts in the beliefs, thoughts, or intentions of speakers. As Nelson explains, meaning can be distinguished from the intentions of the speaker, or his or her beliefs: "practices might have expressive content in a way that is not solely a function of our beliefs" (Nelson 1998, 178). Nelson makes this point in order to counter a potential argument against the expressivist objection. According to this anti-expressivist position, a prospective parent might argue that a choice to selectively terminate does not express a negative message about disabilities because no such message was intended. Such a person might claim that she chose selective termination, for instance, because she was concerned about the economic impact on her family of raising a child with a disability. According to the Wittgensteinian theory of meaning, selective termination might nonetheless convey a negative message about disabilities regardless of what the prospective parent intended. The choice to selectively terminate might play a role in a language game whose outcome is a negative message about disabilities.

A further aspect of a Wittgensteinian theory of meaning is that the systems of rules that determine meaning (language-games) should not be seen as strict and unchanging. Language-games are conventional. The rules of language-games themselves also arise out of our practices, just as the practices that convey meaning based on these rules are part of our conventional activity. These conventional activities in which language games are embedded are what Wittgenstein calls a "form of life" (Wittgenstein [1953] 1997).

To illustrate this theory of meaning, consider an example. Nelson contrasts prenatal testing and termination decisions with the action of raising the confederate flag over the South Carolina State House. In her estimation, flying the flag has an unambiguous racist meaning, regardless of the intentions or beliefs of those who are responsible: "One simply could not say that flying the battle flag over the State House means whatever 'we' want it to mean" (Nelson 1998, 178). Instead of being determined by the intentions of those who raise the flag, the meaning of flying the flag is rather set in place by the historically determined system of symbols in which the confederate flag operates as a representation and endorsement of the practice of slavery. Within the historically determinate form of life of the old South, the flag represents support for the states that fought to preserve slavery. The "language-game" of raising flags and using flags to represent states and armies, determines this meaning. The person who raises the flag on a given day might not have intended to convey a racist message. Nonetheless, the act's participation in this system of symbols embedded in this particular form of life is responsible for the message it conveys.

Though Nelson goes along with the expressivist argument this far by outlining a theory of meaning by which an action can convey a message, she ultimately does not endorse the expressivist position. Nelson argues that the practice of prenatal screening for disabilities, and of selective termination "do not take place against a settled practice of seeing them as expressing what a community is and with what it identifies" (Nelson 1998, 178). According to Nelson, the actions associated with prenatal testing and selective abortion do not take place within a system of symbols that is semantically stable enough to avoid ambiguity. On this view, there is no "language-game" within which the practice of prenatal testing operates that gives it an anti-disability meaning. Because ambiguity is not avoided, Nelson argues, prenatal testing and selective abortion cannot legitimately be seen as expressing any determinate messages.

To contest Nelson's argument, I believe that there is a "settled practice" or set of "language-games" that provides a semantic framework within which the social phenomenon of prenatal testing can be legitimately interpreted as sending negative messages about people with disabilities. This settled practice is medicalization: specifically the medicalization of pregnancy, and the medicalization of disability. Medicalization is the practice of viewing these conditions (pregnancy, disability) through the lens of biomedicine. The medicalization of disability, for instance, takes a category of human difference, and makes the category a subject of medicine. A hallmark of medicalization is the transformation of features of normal human life into pathological states, when these features might otherwise be understood merely as instances of normal human variation, or go unrecognized altogether. Medical discourse and practices thus regard disabilities as problems to which diagnostics, and treatments or interventions should be applied (Conrad 2007). The medical profession has the epistemic authority to dictate what constitutes a normal human body, mind, or genetic code, and what constitutes a departure from normality. According to the medicalized depiction, the problems associated with disabilities inhere in the body of the person himself or herself who has the disability. The cause is within. The solution to these problems is to fix or treat the body. I will argue that just as raising the confederate flag cannot avoid sending a racist message, disability is caught up in a system of screening, diagnostics, technological intervention, and professional expertise that cannot avoid sending the message that the birth of people with disabilities should be avoided.

The medicalized story is not the only way of understanding disability. The medicalization of disability is only one contender among others offering a public understanding of what disability is. For instance, the "social model" of disability is another view (Krahn 2011; Saxton [1998] 2010). According to the social model, disabilities do not inhere in, and are not caused by, features of the person himself or herself, but are instead caused by one's social arrangements and social environment. To use a well-worn example, someone who uses a wheelchair will be disabled by a lack of accessibility features in the built environment, such as ramps. When these disabling features of the social environment and social organization are addressed, disability no longer exists. Stigma and bias directed at people with disabilities are further disabling features of the social environment. According to Marsha Saxton, disability results from "discriminatory attitudes and thoughtless behaviors, and the ensuing ostracism and lack of accommodation" (Saxton [1998] 2010, 122) rather than from the physical or cognitive characteristics of individuals. Those who endorse the social model would improve the lives of people with disabilities by addressing these social causes of disability, rather than fixing their bodies, minds, or genetic codes. One implication of the social model is that disability is not viewed as pathological.

Though the social model is a contender for the public understanding of disability, the medicalized view is dominant. The social model is a minority perspective that has only partial influence on public understanding. The high rates of selective termination for disabilities like Down syndrome are suggestive of the dominance of the medicalized view of this condition. These high rates are more consistent with viewing Down syndrome as a genetic disorder, rather than with viewing society as disordered in its inability to accommodate the needs of people with genetic differences (Lippman 1991). Furthermore, the medicalized view of disability is dominant because powerful actors advance this view. Doctors are the traditional agents of medicalization, and these professionals are influential. Their influence has been joined by the biotechnology industry, large pharmaceutical corporations, and well-funded genetics researchers (Conrad 2007). The industrial actors behind recent advances in prenatal genomics are highly profitable and are able to project the messages needed to promote their products into the medical profession and directly to consumers (Munthe 2015). These messages require that genetic differences associated with disability are seen as pathological so that there is an urgency to their identification in utero. The agents who advance the social model of disability, in contrast, are significantly less influential and command comparatively meagre resources. These agents consist in disability activists, academics, and grass-roots advocacy organizations.

5.6 The Meaning of the Social Phenomenon of Prenatal Testing

In affluent societies, pregnancy is a thoroughly medicalized condition. Prenatal care typically involves technological monitoring virtually from the beginning, including such processes as the confirmation of pregnancy through testing, both at home, or by a health care professional, and the common use of ultrasound to confirm fetal age or the date of conception. Ongoing care throughout pregnancy involves various routine blood tests, weight monitoring, and regular expert surveillance through check-ups. In different ways, pregnant women are also offered advice on diet and lifestyle that has been developed through biomedical expertise. When women give birth in hospitals, babies enter the world in highly technologized environments with associated pharmacological, physical, or surgical means for facilitating their delivery. Even with less medicalized versions of this arc of care, such as midwifery care, the technological biomedical interventions are usually available and waiting in the wings in case anything does not go to plan.

Pregnancy is judged against a standard of normalcy developed by biomedicine (Sherwin 2001). Deviations from the "normal" are handled by further medical interventions or by increased technological surveillance. Within the medicalized context of pregnancy, the dominant understanding of disability is also highly medicalized. Consider, for instance, the definition of Down syndrome provided by the Mayo Clinic:

> Down syndrome is a genetic disorder caused when abnormal cell division results in an extra full or partial copy of chromosome 21. This extra genetic material causes the developmental changes and physical features of Down syndrome.
>
> Down syndrome varies in severity among individuals, causing lifelong intellectual disability and developmental delays. It's the most common genetic chromosomal disorder and cause of learning disabilities in children. It also commonly causes other medical abnormalities, including heart and gastrointestinal disorders (Mayo Clinic 2018).

This definition is meant to be fact-based, clinical, and inoffensive. However, it presents a particular understanding in which people with Down syndrome have all sorts of problems (intellectual and learning disabilities, developmental delays, and medical abnormalities) and these problems are caused by a genetic feature that inheres within the person himself or herself who has Down syndrome. The problem can be found within the person, rather than outside of the person in the social circumstances that make uncommon learning and developmental needs difficult to accommodate (Kaposy 2018).

Against the background of a medicalized understanding of pregnancy and of disability, a pregnant woman who is found to be carrying a fetus with trisomy 21 is a departure from normalcy, and is a candidate for intervention or increased medical monitoring. As Susan Sherwin notes, within the medicalized worldview all pregnancies are seen as potentially high risk problematic pregnancies. Maternity hospitals, for instance, are organized in a way that is poised to respond to unforeseen crisis for any delivery (Sherwin 2001). There is thus a strong biomedical need to identify, during the prenatal stage in as many pregnancies as possible, whether any "problems" exist before they become crises. The expansion and perfection of prenatal genetic screening and diagnostics are a part of this effort to anticipate, identify, intervene, and counter any problems that occur in pregnancy. The very fact that such effort is taken to test for disabilities in pregnancy indicates to the audience of those who would undergo testing that disabilities are negative characteristics that should be eliminated (Thomas 2017; Lippman 1991).

Within the logic of medicalization, medical testing is used to identify diseases, disorders, disabilities, and the like – departures from normal health, as defined by the medical profession. Genetic variations in pregnancy are defined as problems, and problems must be monitored. The purpose of identifying and monitoring problems is to administer a medical or technical solution. Prenatal testing can help identify fetuses that need prenatal interventions like transfusions, or postnatal intensive care access. But in most cases, in the prenatal period, the only solution currently available for avoiding the identified "problem" of disability is to terminate the pregnancy and avoid giving birth.

5.6.1 Examples of Medicalization in Action

The processes of medicalization encountered at the level of the prenatal clinic reinforce the view that disabilities are something to be avoided, and thus that disabled children ought not to be born. Gareth Thomas's in-depth study of Down syndrome screening at clinics in the UK highlights several features of the process of medicalization that contribute to this message (Thomas 2017). Thomas's work shows how practices in the delivery of prenatal care convey negative messages about disability. Though these examples would likely not occur in every clinic, they illustrate how medicalization can be actualized in the clinic in a way that favours a certain view of disabilities. According to Thomas, "Down's syndrome is imbued with negativity … as something which *can* and *should* be detected and, if a diagnosis is established, as something which constitutes a reason for terminating a pregnancy" (Thomas 2017, 177).

For instance, midwives in the clinics Thomas studied frequently referred to Down syndrome as a "risk", a "problem", or as an "abnormality" (Thomas 2017, 131). Language like this conveys the direct impression that Down syndrome is something that prospective parents ought to avoid. Thomas also documents several instances in which sonographers informed prospective parents that if they received a positive result on a Down syndrome screening test, amniocentesis would be "advised" (Thomas 2017, 79). The message here is that according to professional medical opinion, Down syndrome is something important to diagnose, or a condition with a dire impact. The language used to describe Down syndrome or the screening process carries powerful messages about disabilities.

Thomas's study shows furthermore that Down syndrome is pathologized in offhand ways by the screening process. In the clinics Thomas studied, little time was allocated to pre-screening counselling, leading to the impression that screening for Down syndrome was a routine procedure in which pregnant women would normally and obviously want to participate (Thomas 2017). Furthermore, during the limited counselling time provided, there was a lack of discussion about Down syndrome itself, and the screening test for this condition was offered in conjunction with tests for "rubella, HIV, syphilis, rhesus disease, sickle-cell disease, thalassemia, hepatitis B/C" (Thomas 2017, 132). The combination of the lack of discussion about Down syndrome, and the inclusion of Down syndrome among these diseases, surely conveys the message that it is obvious that one should screen for Down syndrome. In such a context, a patient can easily assume that there is no need to discuss Down syndrome because, like syphilis, it is something that a parent would want to avoid.

The organization of Down syndrome screening in such clinics was set up to lead to termination should the fetus be diagnosed with Down syndrome. For instance, in one clinic, pregnant women who received a positive screening result for Down syndrome were pre-booked for an amniocentesis (and were told about this pre-booked appointment) even before the pregnant women had established for themselves that they wanted this procedure, and before they had given their informed consent (Thomas 2017, 117). The official reason for this practice was the administrative necessity of managing appointment bookings within the short window of time between screening, diagnostic testing, and the availability of termination. But even so, these procedures presuppose that there is an urgency to identify fetuses with Down syndrome so that a termination can be scheduled in a short period of time.

A further example of this feature of medicalization is the practice of "reflex testing" with NIPT as a secondary screening test. Reflex testing is the practice of taking two samples of blood from pregnant women so that if the first sample provides a positive result for a trisomy like Down syndrome on a less-accurate screening test, the second sample can automatically be used for more accurate NIPT (Ravitsky 2017; Wald et al. 2017). Some clinicians have recently begun the practice (Wald et al. 2017). In such instances it may be unclear whether the women have consented to the secondary screening test. The assumption behind such testing is that pregnant women would obviously want to know whether their fetuses have a disabling condition so that they can take action based on this information. This assumption makes sense only if it is first assumed that disabilities are something that prospective parents ought to avoid.

5.6.2 *The Logic of Medicalization*

Returning to Nelson's analogy, the Confederate flag cannot mean anything we want it to mean. Meaning is held in place by a history of practices, by the language-games in which an act plays a role. Similarly, the medicalization of pregnancy and the medicalization of disability provide a stable set of meanings to the social phenomenon of prenatal testing. The set of practices associated with medicalization hold a particular meaning in place. These practices include the procedural steps that begin with surveillance in pregnancy, and screening tests, which lead to diagnostic testing, and ultimately to treatment, which in the case of prenatal testing is the termination of pregnancy. These work processes of screening, diagnosis, and treatment follow a commonplace logic of medical care. According to this logic, the genetic differences identified as disabilities are pathological—something to be avoided in pregnancy. The message is that people with such differences should not be born. Medicalization inhibits us from making these processes mean whatever we want them to mean.

The vast sums of money devoted to perfecting the prenatal identification of genetic differences make sense within this logic of medicalization in which disabilities are pathologies to be avoided. Test development companies obsessively market their products as providing early detection (e.g. LifeLabs Genetics 2018). The main purpose of early detection is to enable fetal diagnosis early enough in pregnancy for termination to be available, since many jurisdictions limit access to abortion past a point sometime in the second trimester of pregnancy.

The expansion of prenatal testing through professional guidelines that extend testing programs so that they include all pregnant women makes sense within this pathologized depiction of disabilities. According to the medicalized understanding of disability, it is necessary to avoid the birth of people with these differences whenever possible, so prenatal testing must be made available to everyone. Selective termination rates are high because disabilities are understood as pathological.

The clinical routinization of prenatal testing likewise makes sense within this medicalized framework. Within this way of thinking it is simply obvious that prospective parents would want to avoid the birth of children with genetic disabilities, so there is no great impetus to gain proper informed consent. Since a medicalized understanding of disability is dominant in our culture, when people with disabilities witness these aspects of the social phenomenon of prenatal testing, it is legitimate for them to interpret this phenomenon as expressing the message that people like them should not have been born.

5.7 Autonomy as an Outcome Rather than Termination

Some will dispute this account and claim that there is an alternate meaning that can be attributed to the medical processes of prenatal testing. According to this alternate interpretation, the endpoint of the screening and diagnostic process is not the termination of pregnancy, but the autonomous choice of the pregnant woman to either terminate or to continue the pregnancy. The autonomous choice to refuse prenatal screening or diagnostic testing is also available to the pregnant woman. Prenatal testing procedures thus support autonomous choice, one might claim, and medicine is agnostic about the social worth of people with disabilities.

But the very fact that there is prenatal testing *at all* for disabilities, and millions of dollars poured into the development of better tests, suggest something other than agnosticism and support for autonomous choice. Clearly disability is not perceived as a mere difference by the actors who advance these interests. The social phenomenon of prenatal testing has not developed over decades as a way of identifying mere differences in the fetus. Disabilities are clearly perceived as something pathological. The belief that prenatal testing is meant to support autonomous choice is consistent with a belief that a child with a disability is full of problems about which prospective parents should at least be warned. In contrast, the medical profession finds it acceptable to leave mere differences up to chance. For instance, when there is a technological advance, such as prenatal whole-genome sequencing, that would enable prospective parents to pick and choose babies according to traits such as eye-colour or hair-colour, choruses of opposition rise up against "designer babies". Enabling prenatal choices about disabilities engenders very little opposition. There is comparatively more ethical disquiet about the prospective development of prenatal genetic tests for traits perceived to be "neutral".

The depiction of prenatal testing as supporting autonomous choice, rather than leading to selective termination, actually fixes the same messages about disability into place. The all-important mandate to support autonomous choice in reproduction can be read as a duty to warn prospective parents about the consequences of choosing to continue their pregnancies. Choices that are perceived to be unorthodox or potentially harmful invite increased scrutiny. Prenatal testing is a form of increased scrutiny over choices in pregnancy.

As an analogy, we respect the autonomy of people who choose to go back-country skiing, who scuba dive with sharks, go skydiving, or who stay in town during a hurricane. But we make sure that their choices are informed. We convey the message that, "this could be really bad for you, are you really sure you want to do this?" These analogies show that the process of scrutiny and warning is consistent with respecting autonomy. Orthodox choices, in contrast, invite little or no scrutiny. The routinization of prenatal testing, and the expansion of categories of pregnant women eligible for new forms of prenatal testing, suggest that in the medicalized worldview, pregnant women ought to know whether they are carrying a fetus with a disability. The orthodox choice is to undergo prenatal testing. Even though prenatal testing supports autonomous choice, the underlying logic of medicalization still conveys the unavoidable message that people with disabilities should not be born. To swim against the current of orthodoxy and instead choose to bring a child with a disability into the world requires being first met with warnings and scrutiny about the supposed harm that this choice could bring.

5.8 Conclusion

I have argued that the expansion of prenatal genomics, as embodied by the social phenomenon of prenatal testing, sends the message that people with disabilities ought not to have been born. I began by outlining a few disability-based objections to the expansion of prenatal genomics that focus on the potential consequences for people with disabilities of this expansion. From there, I developed an argument in support of the expressivist position. According to the argument, the social phenomenon of prenatal testing sends this negative message about people with disabilities.

The social phenomenon of prenatal testing, as I have defined it, includes the actions of a variety of agents and organizations, such as prospective parents, clinicians, prenatal test development companies, health system decision-makers, and professionals who create clinical practice guidelines. To address the question of how the actions of such a disparate set of actors could convey a univocal message about disability, I pointed out that all of these actions are unified by the overarching medicalization of pregnancy, and the medicalization of disability.

The logic of medicalization provides a Wittgensteinian "language-game" within which all of the actions that contribute to the social phenomenon can be seen as expressing a common message. According to Wittgenstein's theory of meaning, the rules of language-games are not abstract and immutable universal truths. These rules arise out of our practices. Our language games derive from what Wittgenstein calls our "form of life". We can judge the meaning conveyed by a practice such as prenatal testing by attending to the background form of life within which the practice is historically entrenched. As we have seen, the social phenomenon of prenatal testing participates in the logic of medicalized screening and diagnostic tools designed to eliminate disease. NIPT is a screening tool. Such tools are used by the medical profession to eliminate pathology. In this case, the "pathology" in question is genetic difference. Within the context of this dominant set of medicalized practices, it is straightforward to believe that the social phenomenon of prenatal testing sends the message that people with these genetic differences should not be born.

People with disabilities are therefore justified when they believe that the expansion of prenatal genomics conveys negative messages about them and their lives. The disruption of these negative messages would require the rejection of the medicalization of disability, and of pregnancy, by the wider culture, and would require questioning the social value of the technological tools that enable us to reduce the number of people with genetically-based disabilities in our communities.

References

Aymé, S. 2016. If rare diseases are so rare, why do they matter? *On Biology*. https://blogs.biomedcentral.com/on-biology/2016/02/29/if-rare-diseases-are-so-rare-why-do-they-matter/. Accessed 22 June 2018.

Baylis, F. 2017a. Gene editing: Where should we draw the line? *Impact Ethics*. https://impactethics.ca/2017/10/25/gene-editing-where-should-we-draw-the-line/. Accessed 26 Feb 2018.

Baylis, F. 2017b. Genome editing of human embryos broadens ethics discussions. *The Conversation*. http://theconversation.com/genome-editing-of-human-embryos-broadens-ethics-discussions-84888. Accessed 15 Feb 2018.

Benn, P., K.J. Curnow, S. Chapman, S.N. Michalopoulos, J. Hornberger, and M. Rabinowitz. 2015. An economic analysis of cell-free DNA non-invasive prenatal testing in the US general pregnancy population. *PLoS One* 10: e0132313.

Boyd, P.A., M. Loane, E. Garne, et al. 2011. Sex chromosome trisomies in Europe: Prevalence, prenatal detection and outcome of pregnancy. *European Journal of Human Genetics* 19: 231–234.

Canadian Down Syndrome Society. 2014. What prenatal testing means to me. youtu.be/VQp8OJN5Rjk. Accessed 28 Feb 2018.

Conrad, P. 2007. *The medicalization of society: On the transformation of human conditions into treatable disorders*. Baltimore: Johns Hopkins University Press.

Don't Screen Us Out. 2017. Our concerns. http://dontscreenusout.org/. Accessed 26 Feb 2018.

Dondorp, W., G. de Wert, Y. Bombard, et al. 2015. Non-invasive prenatal testing for aneuploidy and beyond: Challenges of responsible innovation in prenatal screening. *European Journal of Human Genetics* 23: 1438–1450.

Goobie, S., and C. Prasad. 2012. XYY syndrome. *eLS: Citable Reviews in the Life Sciences*. https://doi.org/10.1002/9780470015902.a0005157.pub2. Accessed 30 June 2018.

Gyngell, C., and T. Douglas. 2016. Selecting against disability. The liberal eugenic challenge and the argument from cognitive diversity. *Journal of Applied Philosophy* 33(4).

Hofmann, B. 2017. You are inferior! Revisiting the expressivist argument. *Bioethics*, 31 (7): 505–514.

Human Fertilisation and Embryology Authority. 2018. PGD conditions. https://www.hfea.gov.uk/pgd-conditions/. Accessed 28 Feb 2018.

Human Fertilisation and Embryology Authority. 2008. Human Fertilization and Embryology Act 2008, Code of Practice. https://www.legislation.gov.uk/ukpga/2008/22/section/23. Accessed Nov 7 2021.

International Summit on Human Gene Editing. 2015. On human gene editing: International summit statement. https://www.nationalacademies.org/news/2015/12/on-human-gene-editing-international-summit-statement. Accessed 15 Feb 2018.

Grant, K. 2018. The birth of a revolution in prenatal screening. *The Globe and Mail,* 10 Jan 2018. https://www.theglobeandmail.com/life/parenting/new-prenatal-tests-for-parents-gets-mixed-feelings/article37570374/. Accessed 26 Feb 2018.

Kaposy, C. 2013. A disability critique of the new prenatal test for Down syndrome. *Kennedy Institute of Ethics Journal* 23(4): 299–324.

Kaposy, C. 2018. *Choosing Down syndrome: Ethics and new prenatal testing technologies.* Cambridge, MA: MIT Press.

Krahn, T.M. 2011. Regulating preimplantation genetic diagnosis: The case of Down's syndrome.*Medical Law Review* 19: 157–191.

Lantos, J.D. 2016. Trisomy 13 and 18 – treatment decisions in a stable gray zone. *JAMA* 316(4): 396-398.

Learn from Autistics. 2016. Prenatal screening for autism. https://learnfromautistics.com/prenatal-screening-for-autism/. Accessed 27 June 2018

LifeLabs Genetics. 2018. Learn important health information about your baby, earlier. https://www.lifelabsgenetics.com/product/non-invasive-prenatal-testing/. Accessed 22 June 2018

Lippman, A. 1991. Prenatal genetic testing and screening: Constructing needs and reinforcing inequities. *American Journal of Law and Medicine* 17: 15–50.

Löwy, I. 2014. Prenatal diagnosis: The irresistible rise of the "visible" fetus. *Studies in the History and Philosophy of the Biological and Biomedical Sciences* 47: 290–299.

Mansfield, C., S. Hopfer, and T.M. Marteau. 1999. Termination rates after prenatal diagnosis of Down syndrome, spina bifida, anencephaly, and Turner and Klinefelter syndromes: A systematic literature review. *Prenatal Diagnosis* 19: 808–813

Mayo Clinic. 2018. Down syndrome: Symptoms and causes. https://www.mayoclinic.org/diseases-conditions/down-syndrome/symptoms-causes/syc-20355977. Accessed 28 Feb 2018

Munthe, C. 2015. A new ethical landscape of prenatal testing: Individualizing choice to serve autonomy and promote public health: A radical proposal. *Bioethics* 29(1): 36–45.

Natoli, J.L., D.L. Ackerman, S. McDermott, and J.G. Edwards. 2012. Prenatal diagnosis of Down syndrome: A systematic review of termination Rates (1995–2011). *Prenatal Diagnosis* 32: 142–153

Nelson Goff, B.S., N. Springer, L.C. Foote, C. Frantz, M. Peak, and C. Tracy, et al. 2013. Receiving the initial Down syndrome diagnosis: A comparison of prenatal and postnatal parent group experiences. *Intellectual and Developmental Disabilities* 51(6): 446–57.

Nelson, J.L. 1998. The meaning of the act: Reflections on the expressive force of reproductive decision making and policies. *Kennedy Institute of Ethics Journal* 8(2): 165–180

Nuffield Council on Bioethics. 2017. *Non-invasive prenatal testing: Ethical issues.* https://www.gov.uk/government/news/safer-screening-test-for-pregnant-women. Accessed 15 Feb 2018.

Porter, G., and M.K. Smith. 2013. Preventing the selection of "deaf embryos" under the Human Fertilisation and Embryology Act 2008: Problematizing disability? *New Genetics and Society* 32(2): 171–189.

Ravitsky, V. 2017. Choice not "reflex": Routine prenatal screening. *Impact Ethics.* https://impactethics.ca/2017/12/01/choice-not-reflex-routine-prenatal-screening/. Accessed 28 Feb 2018.

Rochman, B. 2017. *The gene machine: How genetic technologies are changing the way we have kids – and the kids we have.* New York: Scientific American / Farrar Strauss and Giroux.

Saxton, M. 2010. Disability rights and selective abortion. In *The Disability Studies Reader*, ed. Lennard J. Davis, 120–132. New York: Routledge

Seavilleklein, V. 2009. Challenging the rhetoric of choice in prenatal screening. *Bioethics* 23(1): 68–77.

Sequenom. 2017. *Screen for more than Down syndrome.* https://www.sequenom.com/uploads/collateral/MaterniT-GENOME-patient-brochure_Rep-1038.pdf. Accessed 15 Feb 2018.

Sheldon, T., and J. Simpson. 1991. Appraisal of a new scheme for prenatal screening for Down's syndrome. *British Medical Journal* 302: 1133–1136.

Sherwin, S. 2001. Normalizing reproductive technologies and implications for autonomy. In *Globalizing feminist bioethics: Crosscultural perspectives*, ed. R. Tong, 96–113. Boulder, CO: Westview Press.

Stein, Z., and M. Susser. 1971. The preventability of Down's syndrome. *HSMHA Health Reports* 86: 650–658.

Stein, Z., M. Susser, and A. Guterman. 1973. Screening programme for prevention of Down's Syndrome. *The Lancet* 301: 305–310.

Summers, A.M., S. Langlois, P. Wyatt, and R.D. Wilson, et al. 2007. Prenatal screening for fetal aneuploidy. *Journal of Obstetrics and Gynaecology Canada* 29(2): 146–161.

Thomas, G. 2017. *Down's syndrome screening and reproductive politics: Care, choice, and disability in the prenatal clinic*. New York: Routledge.

Wald, N.J., W.J. Huttly, J.P. Bestwick, et al. 2017. Prenatal reflex DNA screening for trisomies 18, and 13. *Genetics in Medicine,* 20(8): 825–830.

Waitzman, N.J., P.S. Romano, and R.M. Scheffler. 1994. Estimates of the economic costs of birth defects. *Inquiry* 31(2): 188–205

Wendell, S. 1996. *The rejected body*. New York: Routledge.

Wittgenstein, L. [1953] 1997. *Philosophical investigations*. G.E.M. Anscombe, trans. Cambridge, MA: Blackwell

Wright, D. 2011. *Downs: The history of a disability*. New York: Oxford University Press.

Part III
Voices of Social Sciences and the Humanities

Chapter 6
The Hypothetical Healthy Newborn

Rosemarie Garland-Thomson

Abstract This chapter is an opportunity to conceptualize a narrative figure that is fundamental in the current clinical procreative process. This figure, I suggest, structures the epistemological environment, what I call the arc of knowing, in which parents must exercise patient autonomy. I will call this narrative figure the hypothetical healthy newborn. My explication here of the cultural work of the hypothetical healthy newborn reveals, perhaps clarifies, the moral conflict at the heart of a pregnant woman's dual obligation to her own best interests and the best interest of her future child.

6.1 The Arc of Knowing

This paper is an opportunity to conceptualize a narrative figure that is fundamental in the current clinical procreative process. This figure, I suggest, structures the epistemological environment, what I call the arc of knowing, in which parents must exercise patient autonomy. I will call this narrative figure the hypothetical healthy newborn.[1]

The hypothetical healthy newborn haunts the gathering arc of knowing that accrues throughout the perinatal, prenatal, and postnatal environment. This figure is the goal, the end point, the desired outcome of the medical procreative process that now begins ideally with preconception obstetrical counseling and clinical visits and ends with routine neonatal screening and care. The figure of the hypothetical healthy newborn is a guiding presence for a prospective parent, the entire obstetrical team of clinicians and healthcare workers in the particular obstetrical practice or hospital,

[1] The purpose of this paper in the development of my own project as a bioethicist is twofold: first, to develop an accurate moral rather than a medical vocabulary to discuss procreative bioethics; second, to work toward developing an argument/rationale against eugenic selection that is not anchored in divine authority but rather is conceptualized as a contribution to the common good.

R. Garland-Thomson (✉)
Emory University, Atlanta, GA 30322, USA
e-mail: rgarlan@emory.edu

M. A. Allyse and M. Michie (eds.), *Born Well: Prenatal Genetics and the Future of Having Children*, The International Library of Bioethics 88,
https://doi.org/10.1007/978-3-030-82536-2_6

the prenatal testing counselors and technicians, as well as the cultural institution of medicine itself. The cultural work of this representational figure of the healthy newborn is to structure the relationship that parents as decision-makers develop with the future child as potential person, embryo, and fetus; that is, the gestating being in the procreative process. My concern here, then, is how the figure of a hypothetical healthy newborn affects the way parents carry out the responsibilities of patient autonomy and procreative liberty in relation to their knowledge of this particular unborn person.[2]

The hypothetical healthy newborn follows the concept of the "Hypothetical Blind Man," a long-standing figure in philosophical thought recently explicated by the blind disability studies scholar Georgina Kleege.[3] This illusory blind man occupies a central place in the philosophical thought experiments of Descartes, Diderot, Locke, Molyneux and others as an ideal of pure blindness that functions as an unambiguous opposite to proper persons and, of course, the sighted philosophers. Such a blind man is hypothetical because, in fact, actual people who have never had any vision are rare. Furthermore, all blind people learn about the visual world, understand sighted experience, and navigate a sighted world because we all share life in an ocularcentric culture. So the hypothetical blind man is a fiction, a philosophical control group human subject, through which philosophers speculate about sighted experience. Kleege reveals that the primary function of this epistemological prop is highlighting the importance of sight and eliciting the kind of pity that strengthens gratitude amongst sighted philosophers for the vision they have. What this overdetermined theoretical figure of the blind man in philosophical thought experiments precludes is the opportunity for philosophy and philosophers to understand the shared human experience of "blindness as something besides the absence of sight." (42).

The hypothetical healthy newborn functions similarly as a prop in both the clinical and the bioethical environments. Like the hypothetical blind man, the hypothetical healthy newborn masquerades as a majority figure in human physiology and experience. Just as there are no humans completely innocent of sight, there are no newborns completely innocent of anomaly or the differences that can count in some way as pathology in our clinical understandings of what it means to be human. Just as actual blind people have both cultural and biological experience of sight, actual newborns display a wide range of variation genetically, morphologically, and temperamentally.

Standards of care, hospital policy, medical treatment protocols, idiosyncratic styles of the healthcare practitioners and technicians involved in every individual procreative process determine the institutional relationship to the hypothetical healthy newborn. Through this process, the hypothetical healthy newborn comes to be realized as the goal of the obstetrical patient as she moves through the temporal,

[2] I use here terms such as procreative process, unborn person, and gestating being in order to place this explication of the hypothetical healthy newborn in the context of the parents' imaginative, emotional, and psychological experience of the gestating child about whom they are making decisions in the present and plans for the future. Thus, I have avoided medical terms such as embryo and fetus in favor of terms that conceptualize this liminal figure as a present and future person.

[3] Georgina Kleege, More Than Meets the Eye: What Blindness Brings to Art (New York: Oxford University Press, 2018).

spatial, material, ideological, physiological, and psycho-emotional facets of the procreative enterprise.

My concern here is not with medical treatment, practices, or policies in the procreative process or what any particular live healthy newborn might actually be. Rather I will consider here the *hypothetical* healthy newborn as a representation, an aspirational abstract ideal rendered through a variety of discourses that range from a genetic profile to a morphological image or description, a commercial image, a family member, a productive and valuable citizen, and also to a human seed imagined as destined to manifest as a being with full moral personhood and a high quality of life. These multiple representations in visual, textual, verbal, auditory, mechanical, quantitative, cultural, and imaginative forms collectively gather in this overdetermined haunting of the procreative process. So whereas the representational forms through which we access the image of the hypothetical healthy newborn are flexible and varied, the essential quality of this figure is quite rigid. That essence is "healthy," a quality that has become increasingly quantitatively defined under the growing influence of genomic medicine in defining human personhood. The figure of the hypothetical healthy newborn thus renders procreative women into, according to Silja Samerski, "managers of fetal risk profiles" (2007).

The work of this chapter, then, is to think through the cultural work of representation in knowledge making as it shapes the experience of and decisions made by parents during the routinization of prenatal testing as they move through the procreative process. I must emphasize that I am formulating figures here that have a relation to embryos, fetuses, and other biological elements that obstetrical practice treats but are in fact themselves epistemological narratives. That relationship is a mimetic one in that narratives, both linguistic and imagistic, are taken to represent the reality of the enfleshed being that is gestating and to which the parents have no direct visual and tactile access. It is primarily, then, through the forms of representation that the medicalized procreative process offers them that they know this child. So while the scope of this chapter is limited to the ethics of representation as it structures epistemology, it reaches toward considerations of how knowledge can be harm more than benefit.[4]

---

[4] Studies and rationales are emerging across academic and professional fields arguing that what I am calling here the arc of knowing during the procreative process constitute harm rather than benefit for women. A thorough review and discussion of this bioethical issue is beyond the scope of this paper. Instead, this paper uses the language of the humanities to explicate this arc of knowing. But the next step to follow this paper would be to make the argument that this is more harm than benefit. See, for example, Katie Stoll, "The Routinization of Prenatal Testing and the Erosion of Patient Autonomy," *The DNA Exchange*, November 16, 2017, https://thednaexchange.com/2017/11/16/the-routinization-of-prenatal-testing-and-the-erosion-of-patient-autonomy/; B.A. Bernhardt et al., "Women's Experiences Receiving Abnormal Prenatal Chromosomal Microarray Testing Results," *Genetic Medicine* 15, no. 2 (2013), 139–145; Silja Samerski, "Genetic Counseling and the Fiction of Choice: Taught Self-Determination As a New Technique of Social Engineering," *Signs: Journal of Women in Culture and Society* 34, no. 4 (2009), 735–761; E Garcia, D R M Timmermans, and Evan Leeuwen, "Reconsidering Prenatal Screening: An Empirical Ethical Approach to Understand Moral Dilemmas as a Question of Personal Preferences," *Journal of Medical Ethics*, 35 (2009), 410–414. See also Rosemarie Garland-Thomson, "How We Got to CRISPR: The Dilemma of Being Human," Perspectives in Biology and Medicine 63, no. 1 (2020), 28–43.

In other words, this chapter theorizes the role of the hypothetical healthy newborn in determining a parent's understanding of the particular unborn person they are bringing into the world and into their family through the procreative process. In my initial review of the vast literature about prenatal testing and the ethics of prenatal testing, I have provisionally concluded that the most useful and prevalent information comes from clinical studies and publications, many of which are from the field of genetic counseling and from bioethical philosophy. There is also a great deal of literature in the public conversation, the bioethical literature, and the professional literature that focuses on reproductive liberty. However, what I offer here is a more limited and focused explication from a humanities knowledge perspective and expression and a cultural analysis. My intention is to expand such explications and conclusions in the interest of working toward a more nuanced understanding of the bioethical issues involved from a cultural perspective and one focused on issues of representation and the meaning making function of narrative and knowledge making.

6.2 The Ethical Paradox of a Patient within a Patient

Everyone in the procreative process, from patients to clinicians, has a relationship to the hypothetical healthy newborn figure. I will focus here, however, on the dual role of the mother as agent in determining the emergence of the future person her body gestates. The mother has three forms of agency in this process: first, her body literally shapes the future person during the process of gestation; second, she comes to know the unborn person her body gestates both through her own embodied experience of the procreative process and through medical knowledge of the particular unborn person she gestates; third, in exercising patient autonomy and her reproductive liberty interests, she determines both the shape and vitality of her unborn child.

The emerging yet unborn person gestating in a mother's body will be passively shaped by the figure of the hypothetical healthy newborn. The mother is the agent of this shaping and the gestating person is the recipient of that shaping. It is this conjoined patient undergoing the treatment of the obstetrical process.[5] Continuously throughout this process of gestation, this human-making enterprise, the mother will be determining through the biological process of gestation both the emergent individuality of this future person and at the same time its viability through her own biology and her exercise of patient autonomy in the specific form of reproductive liberty.

This entanglement between the mother and the gestating person is a distinct version of human embodiment in which we have a patient within a patient. The best interests of the mother and the best interests of the gestating being are biologically inseparable, even though medical ethics is obliged to consider them separately. Whereas both the mother and the emergent person are patients, only she has the obligation and the right to exercise autonomy in medical decision-making. The

---

[5] Alice Dreger, *One of Us: Conjoined Twins and the Future of Normal* (Cambridge, MA: Harvard University Press, 2005).

paradox here, of course, is that in exercising her own patient autonomy, she is making medical decisions for herself and for the unborn person she gestates. This dilemma is a version of what bioethicist Erik Parens calls "the parental obligation to shape" and "the parental obligation to accept."[6]

The being that is the future person and at the same time the object of intense scrutiny as it moves through the process of gestation thus has the unclear and contested moral status of being a person and a nonperson at once.

Although all parents have the obligation to make medical decisions for their children, who are not considered competent decision-makers for themselves, in the case of the pregnant woman the medical decisions she makes for herself are inseparable from the medical decisions she is making for her gestating child. The physiological entanglement inherent in pregnancy presents a singular moral situation in regard to the way we reason medical autonomy in cases where a competent adult is charged with making medical decisions for an incompetent person. The parent making medical decisions on behalf of their child can consider either the expressed or recognized best interests of the child and to separate those interests from what they imagine to be their own best interests or the best interests of the family. While this differentiation between the interests and situation of a parent and child may not be complete, the mother and gestating child are physiologically inseparable so that a mother's best interests are entangled in the gestating person's best interests. We have in the United States and most other countries laws that structure this dilemma of medical decision-making. This chapter will not approach the morality of these laws, but will note that the solution to this problem of patient autonomy is to withhold any status of legal personhood from a gestating person until it is born, even when it can survive independently of its mother's body. I recognize, of course, the moral controversy of this clash of personhood interests.

6.3 The Hypothetical Healthy Newborn as Normate Template

Both an unborn child and the future person are experienced and known to the parent as liminal, as existing between recognizable cultural categories. The being gestating in a woman's uterus is at once a person and not a person, their child and not their child. It is a mixture of intangibles for the parent. Medicine names it an *embryo* or *fetus*, not a proper, finished, or legal person. The liminality of this being arises for the parents because it cannot be experienced as we experience or know an actual person, which is through a sensory experience of that person– touching, seeing, hearing that person. Haptic and visual encounters between people cement the relationships we

[6] Suki Finn, "Bun or Bump," Aeon, July 27, 2017, https://aeon.co/essays/is-the-mother-a-container-for-the-foetus-or-is-it-part-of-her; Elly Vintiadis, "The View from Her," Aeon, August 16, 2021, https://aeon.co/essays/is-there-something-special-about-the-way-women-do-philosophy; Erik Parens, "Made to Order," *Aeon,* November 11, 2015, https://aeon.co/essays/can-parents-be-trusted-with-gene-editing-technology

think of as moral personhood.[7] Both the scale and the sensory experience of this being do not conform to our experience of actual persons. This being falls in between the separate component parts of procreation and the newborn person with the full rights and recognition of personhood that we accord living persons. It is at once imaginary and material, at once fiction and truth.

The biological being that will become their future child is thus a liminal being in the cultural environment, which– it can be argued– is the environment, the epistemological landscape, in which the parents experience their unborn child. Liminal is an anthropological concept, which names the epistemological or phenomenological in-between the generally accepted categories or taxonomies that structure particular cultures.[8] Liminal spaces, beings, or experiences provoke anxiety in people because they violate the boundaries of cultural categories and rules, leaving people unsure about how to understand or respond to such liminal phenomena. In response to unsettling liminal phenomena, people construct cultural rituals to help them navigate spatially, temporally, relationally, and psycho-emotionally through these uncertain experiences.[9]

The parent-in-waiting experiences their child in the cultural environment but they know their child in the medical environment. This is so because obstetrical technology has become the primary means of knowing a gestating person. Before these technologies of knowledge yielded the database that defined a gestating person, maternal knowledge gained from the interiority of gestational experience was a primary source for both parents and clinicians. This phenomenological knowledge based on embodied experience is unstable and without much authority in the context of the total environment of the obstetrical clinic where knowledge emanates from what Silja Samerski critically calls "genetic literacy, or more generally, biomedical literacy" (737).

The hypothetical healthy newborn is an infant version of what Aimi Hamraie calls "the normate template." This template is a model of the hypothetical person for whom the built and imagined world is designed.[10] Various influential versions of this normate template predate the current clinical ideal of the hypothetical healthy newborn. Among its predecessors are Leonardo's Vitruvian man, Adolphe Quetelet's Average Man, Le Corbusier's Modulor, and the 1940s anthropometric figues of

[7] Consider here Emmanuel Levinas and Maurice Merleau- Ponty on the importance of sensory knowledge in both the accordance and development of personhood.

[8] See Victor Turner, "Betwixt and Between: The Liminal Period in Rites de Passage", in *The Forest of Symbols* (Ithaca, NY: Cornell University Press, 1967). The disabled anthropologist Robert Murphy uses the theory of liminality to explain the experience of disability in his self-ethnography; see Robert Murphy, *The Body Silent: The Different World of the Disabled*(New York: Norton, 1990).

[9] Anthropologists tend to explicate liminal rituals such as rites of initiation or passage from one stage of life to another. It is more difficult for us to identify liminal anxiety and our cultural responses to it in our own cultural structures. Because the procreation process for us now is so highly structured through the truth discourses of medicine, empiricism, and authority, it may be hard for us to recognize the cultural components of procreation as a system of liminal experiences and cultural rituals.

[10] Aimi Hamraie, *Building Access: Universal Design and the Politics of Disability* (Minneapolis: University of Minnesota Press, 2017). See also Ian Hacking, The Taming of Chance (Cambridge: Cambridge University Press, 1990).

Normman and Norma. As modernity developed from the Renaissance to the modern era, this figure shifted from an aesthetic ideal to a statistical phantom. The hypothetical part of all of these figures is that– like the hypothetical blind man– few actual people conform to these models. So the irony, if you will, or the logical error in the cultural power of such figures is that the aspiration to achieve the contours these figures offer will always fail.

The hypothetical healthy newborn is, then, an inherently unrealized ideal. When it is presented as a goal to mother as patient during the gestational period, it is a promise that cannot be kept. This is so primarily because the hypothetical healthy newborn is abstractly defined by what it is not rather than what it is. The figure is a blank slate from which all indications of pathology have been erased. Another way of considering this is that the hypothetical healthy newborn is an empty signifier. It is a symbolic representation with heavy cultural meaning that has no actual material referent. The processes of testing over the prenatal period have the potential to open up a wider and wider disparity between the achieved goal of producing the hypothetical healthy newborn and the technological and imaginative representation of the actual gestating being. The cumulative medical testing procedures that constitute the arc of knowing the gestating being provide a particularity to the portrait of that being that aims through diagnosis to pry it further and further away from the abstract ideal of that healthy newborn.[11] And at every point in the art of knowing, the emerging particularity of the actual gestating being can become a clinical account made up of "toxic knowledge" that testifies against its acceptability.[12]

6.4 Two Ways of Knowing

The gestating mother experiences an epistemological trajectory, an arc of knowing about her unborn child, as she moves through the phases of obstetrical care from the perinatal planning stage, to the embryonic, fetal, and delivery stages. She will know her unborn child in two ways, one embodied and one representational. In other words, she will know this unborn being through her own experience of touching that being and being touched by that being that is gestating inside her. She will also know this gestating being by way of the authoritative systems of representation that medical technologies provide her during the prenatal period. The embodied way of knowing is phenomenological, where the representational way of knowing is abstract. One way of knowing comes to her from her own being and the other from authoritative clinical discourse. Her own experiential way of knowing, however, has much less authority in the clinical context then the representational way of knowing through medical technology.

[11] The language of research and studies in the field of genetic counseling regularly use diagnostic and prognostic terms such as issue, something wrong, abnormal, blindsided, no-brainer, anomaly, severity, outcomes, disorder, results, findings, risk, health, deletion, and development.

[12] The term "toxic knowledge" comes from B.A. Bernhardt et al., "Women's Experiences Receiving Abnormal Prenatal Chromosomal Microarray Testing Results," *Genetic Medicine* 15, no. 2 (2013), 139–145. See also Allison Werner-Lin, Judith L.M. Mccoyd, Barbara A. Bernhardt, "Actions and Uncertainty: How Prenatally Diagnosed Variants of Uncertain Significance Become Actionable," Hastings Center Report 49, no. 3 (2019), S61–71.

The reason her phenomenological experience of knowing this unborn being has less authority than the clinical knowing is twofold. First and most straightforward is that clinical knowledge has more authority in the clinic than individual personal embodied knowledge. The second reason has to do with the liminal status of an unborn being. The fetus is an exception to our culturally accepted understanding of what it means to be a fully human person. In some ways this is counterintuitive, because of course every full human person was at one point a fetus, even though in our contemporary moment we take the gestating being as an exception in our legal and moral conception of full personhood. Thus the gestating being is not a legal or material person, in the sense that we define human personhood in terms of its visual and haptic availability to us. In other words, a both legal and moral full human person is available to other human persons through the senses, primarily the sense of touch. We know other human beings and recognize their full moral personhood as we experience them through our senses. In the case of a gestating person, this direct sensory validation of personhood is not available to the mother or to any of us. Although the mother is able to haptically experience her unborn child, that sensory relationship to the child is different from the relation that equal moral persons have with one another or that she will have with this child once it is born. The status of moral personhood for both mother and child during pregnancy is, then, an exceptional instance that complicates, perhaps even violates, our cultural understanding of moral personhood as being granted only to human singletons.[13]

What I'm calling representational knowing– that which carries most authority within a clinical environment– has expanded in complexity and authority as medical technologies have made the goal to produce the hypothetical healthy newborn increasingly possible. The array of epistemological technologies now a part of the obstetric standard of care have made this gestational being known in ways that recently complicate the parents' relationship with this liminal being and introduce new processes of decision-making to the ethical landscape of patient autonomy.

In thinking through the cultural work of the hypothetical healthy newborn in the procreative process, it is useful to recognize that the arc of knowing is much more than simply a data set about a particular embryo or fetus. Certainly the obstetrical technologies yield information about the inchoate person who is the co-patient along with the procreative woman. Because these technologies of representation in application have temporal and spatial material dimensions, they are experiences in time and space that create a dynamic multimodal narrative of a developing person in transition from embryo to newborn. These epistemological technologies are understood in the clinical setting as data acquisition methods that include ultrasound/sonogram, maternal blood tests, and direct sampling of placental, fetal or embryonic cells. The application of these technologies is monitored and structured by guidelines from professional organizations such as the American College of Obstetrics and Gynecology as well

[13] The human conditions that challenge this equation of moral personhood and human singleton status are the universal, and thus common, stage of human pregnancy and the very rare human condition of conjoinment. For more on singleton status, see Alice Dreger, *One of Us: Conjoined Twins and the Future of Normal* (Cambridge, MA: Harvard University Press, 2005).

as insurance companies. The data is interpreted through genetic technologies and by clinical experts. A pregnant or perinatal woman as patient experiences these "data acquisition" procedures, however, as events in time and space done with machines to her body with her consent given in a clinical context that encourages her to undergo these experiences. Such medical mechanical procedures yield clinically mediated information that is for her a series of narratives in multiple formats ranging from images to words, texts, and numbers. What she has is a vivid and detailed cumulative portrait compiled over time of a being with a potential human future and distinctive human traits but that is unrecognizably human through her own direct experience. She must, then, imagine this being's full humanity by way of this series of representations. This aggregate representation of a liminal human being is not simply descriptive, but it is diagnostic. In other words, whereas the series of dynamic clinical portraits renders this being in all of its particularity in the now, the purpose of this cumulative representation is to create a much more speculative image of a future human being developing over a lifetime. Such an imaginative task is mediated for a procreative woman by the strong authority of medical interpretation in the context of vulnerability for her as patient. On the basis of these shifting and multimodal representations, she must make decisions about medical treatment for this being, to include terminating its viability.

6.5 Vitality

My explication here of the cultural work of the hypothetical healthy newborn figure reveals, perhaps clarifies, the moral conflict at the heart of a pregnant woman's dual obligation to her own best interests and the best interest of her future child. We might imagine a pregnant woman understanding her own best interests in three ways: first, in terms of her own health, both mental and physical; second, in terms of the needs and intentions she has for the family she is making; third, in terms of the particular being she is gestating. Her moral situation is to balance these interests and obligations. As the pregnancy develops, so too does the phenomenological and representational arc of knowing I have described, structuring the decisions she must make during her pregnancy. As I have noted, the pregnant woman is the decision-making agent in the procreative process, the patient understood as competent and autonomous– legally, medically, and ethically– to make decisions for both herself and the being she is gestating, a liminal being who has no legal status as a person.[14] Hovering above this complex moral situation is the figure of the hypothetical healthy newborn. Its abstract presence creates a triangular relationship among the mother, the actual developing being, and the hypothetical healthy newborn to which representations of the actual gestating being are perpetually compared. The authority of the hypothetical healthy

[14] Again, I will not take up here the moral status of the gestating being, in part because it is the legal and medical status of that being that dictates what can and cannot be done to it in the current medical and legal context of pregnancy.

newborn in the gestational environment interrupts her epistemological relationship with the actual gestating being developing in its own distinctive way into a particular enfleshed being within her body.

Both the pregnant woman and the gestating being have tasks during the procreative period. The woman's task is to shape this gestating being in two ways: first, through the biological process of pregnancy and the curation of her own body during that process; second, through the medical actions she chooses in response to the art of knowing during the process of pregnancy. These decisions are actions consisting of testing, treatment, and/or termination. Her task is understood as a grammatically transitive relationship in which she acts upon the being by carrying out the treatment decisions of procreative liberty. The gestating being's task is understood grammatically as intransitive, it develops according to its own inner logic, what we understand now as its genetic code. As the philosopher Juergen Habermas has it, the woman's task is to *make* a healthy newborn whereas the gestating being's task is to *grow* into itself. When a disparity forms between the woman's task of producing a hypothetically healthy newborn and the revealed contours of the particular gestating being do not conform, the vitality of the gestating being is threatened with termination or normalizing treatment.

Any actual future person must navigate its becoming through the multiple stages of the procreative process in which it becomes known in its distinctive form of being, its particularity. This navigation from conception to birth is the challenge of the emergent human being. Until the recent monitoring of the future person through knowledge technology, the gestating determined its own emergence through sustaining vitality. The diagnosis and prognosis, the knowing and predicting based on medical representations ranging from genetic profiles to morphological images, that is standard obstetrical care now obscure the fundamental task of the emergent person to grow into the particular living being it is becoming during the gestational process. Its moral obligation, if you will, to become its own distinctive living is compromised by what we might consider eugenic gatekeeping directed by the failure of the hypothetical healthy newborn.

We might, then, morally consider vitality as the threshold of full personhood rather than conformity to the ideal of the healthy newborn as a conceptual being stripped of particularity and anomaly. If we were to follow what I might call the vitality threshold rather than the conformity threshold, we might open up a morally welcoming moral environment to human variation in distinctiveness that has passed the test of vitality rather than the tests of normalcy. This would require us to reconceptualize the agency of a gestating being. We would need to understand that being as growing into itself in a way that would sustain its own vitality. So vitality, the capacity to sustain life, would become the threshold for who will be and who will not be in the world. This reconceptualized obstetrical goal would be not a healthy newborn, but simply a living newborn, one prepared to embark on a distinctive life shaped over time and across space by its encounters with world.

Following the logic of this vitality threshold, we may be able to forgo judgment and prognosis about the human shape and function as abstract static phenomena, but rather consider instead how the widest range of human variation can be accommodated by the world we build for ourselves.[15]

We might then take up the moral good of honoring the vastness of human variation that supports vitality, to extend support for human distinctiveness and diversity not just a biological good for the continuation of successful evolution of the human tribe but rather as a moral good in itself, as a fulfillment of a fundamental aspect of our humanness.

[15] An example of this reconceptualization that is beyond the scope of this particular paper, but may serve as an example of using the vitality threshold rather than the normalcy threshold is a recent comment by a mother of the child selected as the 2018 Gerber baby. Lucas Warren, a 1-year-old from Dalton, Georgia who is the first child with Down syndrome to be named a Gerber baby since the contest's start in 2010. "He may have Down syndrome, but he's always Lucas first," said his mother. See Terri Peters, "Meet the First Gerber Baby with Down Syndrome; His Name is Lucas!", *Today.com,* February 7, 2018,
https://www.today.com/parents/2018-gerber-baby-first-gerber-baby-down-syndrome-t122258.

Chapter 7
The Good and the Goal of Pre-conception and Pre-natal Genetic Testing from a Catholic Perspective

Kevin Fitzgerald

Abstract In the United States in particular, one institution that consistently resisted the social momentum to implement eugenic public policies was the Catholic Church. From the Catholic perspective, everyone is worthy, and the focus should be on figuring out how best to care for each individual human being, with access to scarce resources given first to those who need them the most. This chapter addresses the ethical challenge of eugenics and genetic technologies, including preconception and pre-natal genetic testing and genome editing, from the perspective of the medical moral tradition of the Roman Catholic Church. This perspective can contribute to a broad and rich description of human nature and experience, including many types of knowledge and experience, because genetic interventions can and will affect human beings on all levels of their existence.

In this chapter the ethical challenge of eugenics and pre-conception and pre-natal genetic testing will be addressed from the perspective of the medical moral tradition of the Roman Catholic Church.[1] This relevance of exploring this particular religious perspective is two-fold. First, the Catholic Church has an extensive global health care network that must address the local challenges of each community its serves while also providing a medical-ethical decision-making framework that applies consistently and well across the diverse spectrum of human communities and cultures the Church encounters. Therefore, any health system or health care professional might benefit from the Church's two thousand years of experience in trying to bring healing and comfort to the sick. Second, in order to meet this global medical ethics need, the

[1] Sections of this chapter were originally published as "A Catholic Perspective on Human Genome Editing," *National Catholic Bioethics Quarterly*, Vol. 17, No. 1, Spring 2017.

[2] For an outline of the history of Catholic thought on the status of the human embryo, and the impact of the discovery of human ova, see http://www.usccb.org/issues-and-action/human-life-and-dignity/abortion/respect-for-unborn-human-life.cfm (accessed 1/26/19).

K. Fitzgerald (✉)
Creighton University, 2500 California Plaza, Omaha, NE 68178, USA
e-mail: KevinFitzGerald@creighton.edu

M. A. Allyse and M. Michie (eds.), *Born Well: Prenatal Genetics and the Future of Having Children*, The International Library of Bioethics 88,
https://doi.org/10.1007/978-3-030-82536-2_7

Church relies upon its two thousand year old tradition of moral analysis and judgment that is continually updated in light of scientific and technological advances,[2] along with cultural developments, while, at the same time, preserving the fundamental beliefs, values and goals that define the identity of this religious tradition and motivate its healing outreach to the world.

Since part of the identity of the Catholic Church is a call to share its gifts with the world, its medical moral tradition must be both true to its identity, and also accessible in its ethical reasoning to others who are not members of the Church. This accessibility is a requirement because true and complete healing cannot take place without engaging with the patient's life circumstances as well as any physiological problems. Hence, the patient, or the patient's representative, should understand as best as is possible the approach to health care the Catholic institution is committed to providing in order to achieve the best health outcome possible between the health care professionals and the patient.

Though this chapter focuses on only one of the many significant faith traditions around the world, Roman Catholicism, the basic structure used in this chapter of explicating and applying one's fundamental belief system, along with one's ethical reasoning process, to the challenging issue of eugenics and genetic testing is applicable to any health care institution, professional and patient anywhere in the world. Even health care institutions and professionals who might operate from the perspective of allowing the patient to choose whatever intervention they desire, for whatever reason, regardless of current standards of care, have a belief system undergirding that singular patient autonomy approach that they would employ to argue that their patient autonomy only approach is justified.

In more general terms, everyone has a larger world view (grounded in a religious or non-religious tradition, or combination of various traditions) that they use to undergird their reasons for what they decide is good or right, and what is not. When deliberating about how new technological developments might best be used by society, it is always crucial to know and evaluate the larger world view, and ethical reasoning, behind any guidelines or policies an individual or group proposes. This chapter will provide an overview of some of the values and reasoning that undergird a Catholic response to the eugenic issues raised by preconception and prenatal genetic testing.

Before exploring the Catholic perspective regarding preconception and prenatal testing, it is necessary to describe briefly the technologies being addressed. A more thorough examination of the current technological and medical issues involved in this testing can be found in the Executive Summary and the Meeting Summary of the **"Genomic Medicine for Reproductive, Prenatal and Neonatal Health Workshop,"** that was held on April 16–17, 2018, in Bethesda, Maryland, and was sponsored by both the National Human Genome Research Institute (NHGRI) and the Eunice Kennedy Shriver National Institute of Child Health and Human Development (NICHD).[3]

---

[3] Both summaries can be found at https://www.genome.gov/27570856/genomic-medicine-for-reproductive-prenatal-and-neonatal-health/ (accessed 1/26/19).

For the purposes of this chapter, three key technological advances are important to know. First, due to the discovery of fetal cells circulating in the mother's bloodstream, it is now possible to do genetic testing on cells from the fetus by just drawing blood from the mother's arm as might be done for a variety of medical tests. This advance, often called "non-invasive prenatal testing" or NIPT, greatly reduces the risk of harm to the fetus that is present in other testing technologies such as amniocentesis or chorionic villi sampling.[4] The current question regarding NIPT is: whether it can always be as accurate in its results as the older tests have proved to be?

This question leads to the second key technological advance: genome sequencing. The speed, accuracy and cost of sequencing part, or all, of an individual's genome have improved dramatically in the past several years.[5] This advance allows genetic testing to become much more comprehensive than past genetic tests that only looked at specific genes, or sets of genes, or just counted the number of chromosomes looking for abnormalities such as Down Syndrome (which is three chromosome 21 s rather than the common number of two 21 s). While this expanded amount of information may provide a more comprehensive picture of the genetic health of the fetus, it also may reveal unexpected, or even undesired, information—such as the paternity of the fetus, or previously unknown genetic mutations in the parents. In fact, the complexity of the information revealed may also extend beyond the ability of the medical geneticist to understand, potentially causing parents undue anxiety when they hear about genetic differences the fetus has that are of unknown health significance.

This potential anxiety may be further heightened by the third key technological advance—genome editing. This technology is similar to the word editing software used around the world. Instead of changing letters on a page in a document, genome editing technology changes the "letters" of DNA (i.e. the A's, C's, G's, and T's) either to correct a mutation back to a more common letter or set of letters, or to make a new set of letters that are hoped to create an improvement of some kind. Currently there is great interest in the latest genome editing technology, called CRISPR.[6] CRISPR is of great interest because, like genome sequencing technology, it is much less expensive and much easier to use than previous genome editing technologies. However, it is still not completely predictable in its editing of the targeted part of the genome, and so benefits and risks of this technology must be evaluated before it is used to treat embryos and fetuses that have shown known harmful genetic mutations.

In fact, the concern regarding these potential uses of CRISPR among genetic researchers and ethicists was so great that several leading researchers and ethicists published an article in the journal, *SCIENCE*, that concluded:

> At the dawn of the recombinant DNA era, the most important lesson learned was that public trust in science ultimately begins with and requires ongoing transparency and open discussion. That lesson is amplified today with the emergence of CRISPR-Cas9 technology and

---

[4] https://www.genome.gov/27570937/april-17-noninvasive-prenatal-genetic-testing/ (accessed 1/26/19).

[5] https://www.genome.gov/sequencingcosts/ (accessed 1/26/19).

[6] https://www.genome.gov/27569222/genome-editing/ (accessed 1/26/19).

> the imminent prospects for genome engineering. Initiating these fascinating and challenging discussions now will optimize the decisions society will make at the advent of a new era in biology and genetics.[7]

Tragically despite this call for transparency and broad public engagement, which was echoed by many others, a Chinese researcher, Dr. He, shocked the world in November, 2018, when he announced at the Second International Summit on Human Genome Editing in Hong Kong, that he had used CRISPR technology to edit the genomes of two female embryos, who had recently been born in China. The response of the Summit organizing committee summarized well the outrage almost all the participants felt when He made his announcement:

> Even if the [genome] modifications are verified, the procedure was irresponsible and failed to conform with international norms. The organizing committee calls for an ongoing international forum to foster broad public dialogue, develop strategies for increasing equitable access to meet the needs of underserved populations, speed the development of regulatory science, provide a clearinghouse for information about governance options, contribute to the development of common regulatory standards, and enhance coordination of research and clinical applications through an international registry of planned and ongoing experiments.[8]

The committee's statement clearly restates the need for broad public engagement, certainly to foster transparency regarding how genome technologies are being used in research, but also to hear from the public their concerns, fears, hopes and desires regarding how genome technologies should be used in the future. Of course, one can readily conclude that both the Summit committee members, and the SCIENCE article authors, do not expect that each and every adult around the globe will be extensively interviewed to discover what they think, and how they feel, about the potential benefits and risks of genome editing technology. Similarly, broad public engagement regarding the eugenics risks involved in preconception and prenatal genetic testing will not involve surveying even only those adults around the world of reproductive age (however reproductive age may be delineated currently).

One possible starting point for this broad public engagement regarding the use of powerful, and potentially very controversial, technologies is to engage the various large communities around the world that identify themselves as sharing a moral code or world view that arises from their religious or cultural beliefs. While no one can claim empirical evidence of complete homogeneity among any specific large religious community when it comes to all ethical issues, engaging the communities' traditions and documents can reveal the fundamental values and reasoning used to determine how one is to be and act in the world. Hence, this chapter can also be considered one response to these calls for broad public engagement from the biomedical research community.

---

[7] "A prudent path forward for genomic engineering and germline gene modification," by David Baltimore, et al., *SCIENCE,* 3 April 2015, Vol. 348, Issue 6230, pp. 36–8.

[8] http://www.nationalacademies.org/gene-editing/2nd_summit/index.htm (accessed 1/26/19).

7.1 The Catholic Church's Historical Approaches to Health Care and Eugenics

To begin the explication of the Catholic approach to eugenics issues in general, it is useful to first take a historical perspective. In the United States in particular, one institution that consistently resisted the social momentum to implement eugenic public policies was the Catholic Church. This extensive resistance has been documented by Sharon Leon in *An Image of God: The Catholic Struggle with Eugenics*. Leon describes how, during the early twentieth century, the Catholic Church lobbied federal and state governments, and pursued extensive public information campaigns, to protect vulnerable people from eugenic programs, including compulsory sterilization and restrictions on immigration from countries deemed undesirable.

The resistance of the Catholic Church to this public eugenics effort was grounded in two fundamental values. The first value was the importance of good science. Since God created the universe, an accurate scientific grasp of reality should not be in conflict with the care we are all called to give every human being. Hence, the Catholic opposition criticized eugenic science for lacking scientific rigor, concealing blatant ethnic and class biases, and ignoring the importance of social and environmental factors in the development of a person's character. The second value is based in the doctrinal position of personal integrity. From this position, the Church argued that federal or state governments could not violate an innocent individual's bodily integrity, regardless of any alleged biological improvements that might result. In her book's conclusion, Leon states, "The dogged and sustained activism of Catholics made them the primary source of opposition to eugenic sterilization and helped to influence the rejection of negative eugenics initiatives even in places where Catholics did not dominate the public discourse. And at the center of this half-century struggle with eugenics was an unchanging vision of the primacy of all human life."[9]

This unchanging vision of the primacy of all human life remains at the core of the Catholic Church's approach to the global discussion about how to evaluate and employ the advances in preconception and prenatal genetic testing and interventions. To understand the Catholic perspective, it will help to focus on three specific aspects of the Catholic moral tradition: (1) why the Church attaches special significance to the primacy of human life, (2) how the vision of this primacy has developed in response to advances in medical genetic technology, and (3) how the resultant vision of the primacy of human life will be useful, even crucial, in the ongoing global discussion about preconception and prenatal testing and interventions.

One of the four Constitutions written during the Second Vatican Council in the 1960s, *Gaudium et spes* (Joy and Hope), or using its English title - the "Pastoral Constitution on the Church in the Modern World," provides an excellent summary of the Church's vision of the fundamental importance of every human life. At the very beginning of this document, the Church's concern for each human being is made clear:

---

[9] Sharon M. Leon, An Image of God: The Catholic Struggle with Eugenics (Chicago: University of Chicago Press, 2013), 169.

> The joys and the hopes, the griefs and the anxieties of the men of this age, especially those who are poor or in any way afflicted, these are the joys and hopes, the griefs and anxieties of the followers of Christ. Indeed, nothing genuinely human fails to raise an echo in their hearts.[10]

There are several important points to glean from the introduction to *Gaudium et spes*. First of all, the Catholic Church emphasizes that we are all on this journey of life together. Therefore, we need to be in constant communication to find the best ways to bring fulfillment to each life around the world, especially to the poor and afflicted. For Catholics, this global solidarity comes from embracing Christ's mission—the salvation of all humankind. This mission is to be continually worked out in the here and now, addressing the opportunities and challenges of each age in a way that reaches out to everyone in the world, not just members of the Catholic Church, and fosters true human fulfillment for each person on our shared journey toward ultimate fulfillment in God's love.

Later in this same document, the Church expands on the need to remain relevant to the current state of the world by emphasizing the fundamental interdependence of all peoples in the technological age of the 1960s:

> One of the salient features of the modern world is the growing interdependence of men one on the other, a development promoted chiefly by modern technical advances. Nevertheless brotherly dialogue among men does not reach its perfection on the level of technical progress, but on the deeper level of interpersonal relationships... Respect and love ought to be extended also to those who think or act differently than we do in social, political and even religious matters. In fact, the more deeply we come to understand their ways of thinking through such courtesy and love, the more easily will we be able to enter into dialogue with them. . . . Since all men possess a rational soul and are created in God's likeness, since they have the same nature and origin, have been redeemed by Christ and enjoy the same divine calling and destiny, the basic equality of all must receive increasingly greater recognition.[11]

Again, several key points can be found in these sections of *Gaudium et spes*. Though technology is, in a sense, shrinking the world and bringing all peoples closer together, real human closeness requires more than just technological connection. It requires that people acknowledge and value their shared human nature in each human being they encounter. This does not mean that we ignore our differences and disagreements. Instead, recognizing each individual's worth helps each of us learn from our differences in order to gain a better understanding and appreciation both of human diversity and of the need for forgiveness. In fact, the call to affirm the presence of Christ in each person is so strong in the Christian tradition that a Christian is challenged to love and forgive even those who declare themselves enemies and who intend to do harm to Christians. This radical call to love all others—rooted in the actions of Christ during his own ministry, suffering, and execution—is the key element behind the Catholic Church's advocacy on behalf of those threatened by eugenic policies, as well as its emphasis on avoiding any implementation of genetic technology that would selectively harm or eliminate human beings whom others judge to be unworthy of continuing to live as they are.

---

[10] Vatican Council II, Gaudium et spes (December 7, 1965), nn. 1–3.

[11] Ibid., nn. 23, 28–29.

This radical stance of caring for all those who are in need, no matter their circumstances or their attitude toward the Catholic Church, was further institutionalized in 1985 by Pope St. John Paul II's apostolic letter *Dolentium hominum*, which established the Pontifical Commission for the Apostolate of Health Care Workers (later, the Pontifical Council for Pastoral Assistance to Health Care).[12]

This new pontifical commission was to facilitate, from the institutional center of the Church, the fundamental goals all Catholics were to be pursuing in their own ways. If we are to love others as Christ did, then special attention had to be given to those who are suffering and in need. To achieve this goal required an institutional commitment to support health care. That commitment required supporting and enhancing healing that is not merely physiological but also mental and spiritual.

Hence, on both the individual and the institutional levels of the Church, healing can always be made available, even as a patient is dying. Attention to anxiety, depression, and pain can significantly benefit a person even when he is close to death. The overall goal of the Church in caring for those in need is to heal as Christ did—bringing another human being whatever wholeness and fulfillment are possible primarily through loving care, assisted by whatever technology can provide. This approach is consistent with evidence-based medicine, as it has been widely established that patients who feel connected, cared for, and supported do better no matter the medical technology employed.[13]

7.2 Moral Approaches to Genetic Technologies

Among Church documents, *Dignitas personae* most directly addresses genetic interventions:

> For a moral evaluation the following distinctions need to be kept in mind. *Procedures used on somatic cells for strictly therapeutic purposes are in principle morally licit.* Such actions seek to restore the normal genetic configuration of the patient or to counter damage caused by genetic anomalies or those related to other pathologies. Given that gene therapy can involve significant risks for the patient, the ethical principle must be observed according to which, in order to proceed to a therapeutic intervention, it is necessary to establish beforehand that the person being treated will not be exposed to risks to his health or physical integrity which are excessive or disproportionate to the gravity of the pathology for which a cure is sought. The informed consent of the patient or his legitimate representative is also required.
>
> The moral evaluation of *germ line cell therapy* is different. Whatever genetic modifications are effected on the germ cells of a person will be transmitted to any potential offspring. Because the risks connected to any genetic manipulation are considerable and as yet not fully controllable, *in the present state of research, it is not morally permissible to act in*

[12] John Paul II, *Dolentium hominum* (February 11, 1985), nn. 1–2.

[13] For examples both in preventive and critical care medicine, see "Improved Outcomes Start with Patient Engagement," HealthTrust, October 14, 2015, http://healthtrustpg.com/; and Judy E. Davidson et al., "Clinical Practice Guidelines for support of the Family in the Patient-Centered Intensive Care Unit: American College of Critical Care Medicine Task Force 2004–2005," Critical Care Medicine 35.2 (February 2007): 605–622, https://doi.org/10.1097/01.

> *a way that may cause possible harm to the resulting progeny. . . . The question of using genetic engineering for purposes other than medical treatment also calls for consideration.* Some have imagined the possibility of using techniques of genetic engineering to introduce alterations with the presumed aim of improving and strengthening the gene pool. Some of these proposals exhibit a certain dissatisfaction or even rejection of the value of the human being as a finite creature and person. Apart from technical difficulties and the real and potential risks involved, such manipulation would promote a eugenic mentality and would lead to indirect social stigma with regard to people who lack certain qualities, while privileging qualities that happen to be appreciated by a certain culture or society; such qualities do not constitute what is specifically human. This would be in contrast with the fundamental truth of the equality of all human beings which is expressed in the principle of justice, the violation of which, in the long run, would harm peaceful coexistence among individuals. Furthermore, one wonders who would be able to establish which modifications were to be held as positive and which not, or what limits should be placed on individual requests for improvement since it would be materially impossible to fulfil the wishes of every single person. Any conceivable response to these questions would, however, derive from arbitrary and questionable criteria. All of this leads to the conclusion that the prospect of such an intervention would end sooner or later by harming the common good, by favouring the will of some over the freedom of others.[14]

This extended quotation highlights several important aspects of the Catholic moral tradition. The benefits of a procedure must be proportionately greater than the risks it poses to health or physical integrity, so one should not use genetic testing or interventions for anything other than serious medical purposes. Since germline interventions present risks to future generations, they require a level of safety that has not been demonstrated yet and must not involve procedures, such as IVF, that destroy human lives (i.e. embryos). However, therapeutic modifications to germline cells might not be ruled out if adequately safe procedures and desired beneficial outcomes can be obtained. Finally, the use of genetics to select among human beings who shall live and who shall not, or to enhance or change human nature to create supposedly superior beings, is rejected on the basis of the same reasoning that inspired the Church to resist the eugenics movement of the twentieth century. By purposefully attempting to select or create individuals who are considered more valuable or desirable than others promotes a fundamental discrepancy in the valuation of different human beings that violates the Christian vision of the primacy of the equality of all human lives and harms the common good of human society. Considering the horrendous human destruction to which such attitudes have led and continue to lead the human family, the Catholic Church is staunchly opposed to the use of any technology that fosters such attitudes. Instead, the Catholic Church reiterates its emphasis on caring for people where and as they are. From the Catholic perspective, everyone is worthy, and the Catholic tradition clearly includes all human beings from the time of their organismal initiation, that is, almost always conception, to the time of their organismal dissolution, or death. In other words, the focus should be on figuring out how best to care for each individual human being, with access to scarce resources given first to those who need them the most.

---

[14] Congregation for the Doctrine of the Faith, Instruction Dignitas personae, On Certain Bioethics Questions (September 8, 2008), nn. 26–27, original emphasis.

Accepting this Catholic standard of universal care does not necessarily clarify what kind of help we should offer to whom and when. Here again, discerning the appropriate genomic intervention requires a complex yet balanced understanding of individual, community, and species health. This, in turn, demands a comprehensive, integrated, and dynamic framework for understanding human nature and health in order to keep up with both the rapid pace of scientific discovery and the diverse global responses to it.

In earlier works, I have explained at length the advantages of employing a more dynamic and integrative framework in our evaluation of technologies such as human genome editing,[15] so here I will only summarize the elements of this paradigm that pertain to the best use of biotechnologies in the twenty-first century.

To truly understand who we are as a species and who we aspire to become, we need to reflect on all the different fields of inquiry that inform our understanding of ourselves, such as philosophy, theology, law, economics, history, sociology, psychology, literature, the fine arts, political science, and the natural sciences. This broad scope of reflection will need to be balanced as well as inclusive. In other words, each discipline should be approached as a relatively equal partner in this critical effort, since the consequences of employing powerful biotechnologies will be felt in all dimensions of human existence. This comprehensive and integrated approach is deeply rooted in the Catholic intellectual tradition, as exemplified by Pope Benedict XVI in his encyclical letter *Caritas in veritate:*

> This means that moral evaluation and scientific research must go hand in hand, and that charity must animate them in a harmonious interdisciplinary whole, marked by unity and distinction. The Church's social doctrine, which has "*an important interdisciplinary dimension,*" can exercise, in this perspective, a function of extraordinary effectiveness. It allows faith, theology, metaphysics and science to come together in a collaborative effort in the service of humanity.[16]

We see again in this encyclical the theme of the unity of creation and the ways in which we can better understand creation, and our human fulfillment within it, by bringing together the various ways that we know reality. As we work together to bring about our fulfillment within creation, both as individuals and as a species, our integrated knowledge can lead to actions that incorporate the different dimensions of our lives into a common good for all people. This argument for the integration of knowledge and action for the common good is reemphasized by Pope Francis in his apostolic exhortation *Evangelii gaudium*, On the Proclamation of the Gospel in Today's World. Looking particularly at the section titled "Dialogue between Faith, Reason and Science," we find,

> Dialogue between science and faith also belongs to the work of evangelization at the service of peace. Whereas positivism and scientism "refuse to admit the validity of forms of knowledge other than those of the positive sciences," the Church proposes another path, which calls for a

[15] Kevin T. FitzGerald, "The Need for a Dynamic and Integrative Vision of the Human for the Ethics of Genetics," in Genetics, Theology, and Ethics, ed. Lisa Sowle Cahill (New York: The Crossroad, 2005).

[16] Benedict XVI, Caritas in veritate (June 29, 2009), n. 31, original emphasis.

> synthesis between the responsible use of methods proper to the empirical sciences and other areas of knowledge such as philosophy, theology, as well as faith itself, which elevates us to the mystery transcending nature and human intelligence.... All of society can be enriched thanks to this dialogue, which opens up new horizons for thought and expands the possibilities of reason.[17]

Critics respond that these Catholic arguments assume the relevance of including religious experience in public discourse. Although often raised, this criticism is readily addressed on strictly secular grounds, because religious perspectives must be included in any framework that would adequately undergird a global deliberation. I have presented one such argument in previous publications.[18] Its key elements are that (1) flawed epistemological reasoning is behind the claims that scientific knowledge is the only type that should be incorporated into a framework that judges the proper use of biotechnologies, and (2) we need a broad and rich description of human nature and experience, because genetic interventions can and will affect human beings on all levels of their existence. From these two points alone, one can establish the appropriateness of including wisdom from religious traditions, along with many other types of knowledge and experience, in any system of global deliberations.

One can also look at the outcomes that occur from pursuing other approaches to decision-making regarding preconception and prenatal genetic testing and interventions. One decision-making approach that has been widely embraced around the world in the past several decades argues that a patient, or parents, or a legal guardian should make whatever treatment decisions they think are best as long as they can afford the treatment. While this method has certain appealing features—in particular, the simplicity of allowing people to make their own choices for themselves and their children—recent global experience with the use of prenatal diagnostic technologies for sex-selective abortions gives clear evidence of the social problems that can arise from this approach.

Currently, it is widely acknowledged that prenatal sex selection has significantly unbalanced the male–female ratios in China and India, the two most populous nations in the world.[19] However, it is probably much less well known that this problem is also present in other nations around the world and in some populations in the United States.[20] While this situation raises major societal, ethical, and policy issues regarding the use of prenatal diagnosis for sex selection, it also indicates the need to develop ethical and policy approaches to all preconception and prenatal genetic testing and intervention that can balance individual and community goods and goals, especially when the individual and community goals conflict.

To achieve this balanced and inclusive approach extensive public engagement will be required, as has been recognized in the scientific community as cited above.

---

[17] Francis, Evangelii gaudium (November 24, 2013), n. 242.

[18] FitzGerald, "The Need for a Dynamic and Integrative Vision," in Cahill, *Genetics, Theology and Ethics*.

[19] Anna Higgins, "Sex-Selection Abortion: the Real War on Women," American Reports Series, Charlotte Lozier Institute, April 13, 2016, https://lozierinstitute.org/sex-selection-abortion-the-real-war-on-women/ (accessed 1/26/19).

[20] Ibid.

Such an engagement will also draw attention to the marginalized and outcast, whose voices are often not heard in global technological discussions. This kind of public engagement resonates with the emphasis Pope Francis has placed on the Catholic mission of caring for those most in need, which actually benefits all people:

> For the Church, the option for the poor is primarily a theological category rather than a cultural, sociological, political or philosophical one. God shows the poor "his first mercy." . . . We need to let ourselves be evangelized by them.[21]

Though Francis proclaims the theological basis for the Church's strong stance on giving preference to the needs of the poor, he also intimates that the insights into our human condition, which are illustrated in the experiences of the poor, are available for all to see. These are insights that all of us would miss if we choose to ignore or deny the value of their lives and experiences.

7.3 Conclusion

Our world is entering a new age of genetic and genomic information and intervention, which has the potential to impact everyone on the planet significantly, for good or for ill. Scientists and researchers around the globe have acknowledged the need to reach out to the general public to engender a discussion regarding which goods people wish to pursue, and which harms they most wish to avoid. History also provides incentive for this global public engagement that we might avoid repeating the horrors of past eugenic movements.

This global public engagement project is enormous both in its size and its complexity. However, certain areas of possible intervention raise the potential for both tremendous good and harm. Pre-conception and pre-natal genetic testing and intervention are such areas. As such, they have been the focus of this chapter and this book. Surveying each adult on the planet regarding what would be good to pursue and what should be avoided in these areas presents mammoth challenges. On way to circumvent this obstacle would be to start by engaging various cultural and religious communities with large numbers of members who share strong values and commitments that can clearly be applied to these areas of genetic technology. The Catholic Church is one such group that has applied its rigorous, two thousand year old, moral tradition to this topic and has published reflections, conclusions, and hopes regarding how this powerful technology might best serve the good of all people, especially the most vulnerable and needy.

The goal of this chapter was to present how the Catholic Church has reasoned its way to the positions it has taken so far regarding pre-conceptual and pre-natal testing and possible medical interventions using the tools of genome editing technology. The hope of this chapter is that this presentation will facilitate and encourage a truly inclusive global dialogue regarding these technologies and the good ends to which we all can agree to use them.

---

[21] Francis, Evangelii gaudium, n. 198.

Chapter 8
Pathways to Affluence: Socioeconomic Incentives in Prenatal Testing and Abortion

Marsha Michie and Megan A. Allyse

Abstract In this chapter we discuss the ways in which a 'healthy' pregnancy is frequently seen as a more worthwhile pregnancy—and, by extension, evidence of maternal success—while deviation signals the pregnant woman's failure. We argue that, as prenatal screening has continually expanded, so, too, has womens' perceived duty to pre-emptively assess the value of their future child as an individual and as a productive citizen. The underlying assumptions of such calculations, how they have been mobilized to promote universal prenatal genetic screening, and what they reveal about society's perceptions of the roles and duties of potential mothers as arbiters of entry into human society, is the topic of this chapter.

8.1 Introduction

Since its inception, prenatal screening and testing has raised concerns that assessing the health of the fetus corresponds, whether directly or indirectly, with judgments regarding the value of a future child. In a society in which mothering is the hallmark of ideal womanhood, these judgments about the fetus also reflect back upon the woman who carries it. In this chapter we discuss the ways in which a 'healthy' pregnancy is frequently seen as a more worthwhile pregnancy—and, by extension, evidence of maternal success—while deviation signals the pregnant woman's failure. We argue that, as prenatal screening has continually expanded, so, too, has womens' perceived duty to pre-emptively assess the value of their future child as an individual and as a productive citizen. In particular, narratives of prenatal deviation from healthy norms have often invoked decision-making centered on the cost of future individuals

M. Michie (✉)
Department of Bioethics, Case Western Reserve University, 10900 Euclid Ave., Cleveland, OH 44106-4976, USA
e-mail: marsha.michie@case.edu

M. A. Allyse
Program in Biomedical Ethics Research, Mayo Clinic, 4500 San Pablo Road, Jacksonville, FL, USA

M. A. Allyse and M. Michie (eds.), *Born Well: Prenatal Genetics and the Future of Having Children*, The International Library of Bioethics 88,
https://doi.org/10.1007/978-3-030-82536-2_8

perceived to be physically or mentally imperfect, whether this cost is conceptualized as psychosocial burden or, more concretely, as financial burden. As we will see below, entire reports have been devoted to specifying the precise cost of a child born with specific conditions, itemizing the loss to society of an individual's estimated productivity over the lifecourse. The underlying assumptions of such calculations, how they have been mobilized to promote universal prenatal genetic screening, and what they reveal about society's perceptions of the roles and duties of potential mothers as arbiters of entry into human society, is the topic of this chapter.

8.2 Responsible Motherhood and Its Obligations

We begin with the "good" mother. Long a major figure in both psychoanalytic literature and feminist scholarship, the "good" mother has been refigured in contemporary neoliberal discourses of reproduction as the "responsible" mother. Previously appraised on her childrearing decisions after a socially legitimated birth, a mother must now be "good" from the very moment of conception—and even before. While pregnant women are now judged for virtually any choice they make—including bodily activity, environmental exposures, and consumption of both the physical and economic varieties—on the assumption that the welfare of their future child should always take priority, here we are mainly concerned with the ways in which women's decisions about fetal testing and its resulting information are invested with moral value.

Over twenty-five years ago, Shari Thurer declared that "the concept of the good mother is continually reinvented. Each age and each society defines her anew, in its own terms with its own restrictions and expectations." (Thurer 1993), p.519) Similarly, Molly Ladd-Taylor and Lauri Umansky note that what constitutes a "bad" mother has evolved over the last century:

> In the 1920s, a "bad" mother raced to pick up her baby when he cried. Babies were to be left alone in their cribs for several hours a day, not overstimulated by too much cuddling, bouncing, or noise. ... By the 1980s, bestselling author Penelope Leach assured mothers that they could not spoil a baby. ... Now only "bad" mothers meted out solace by the clock. (Ladd-Taylor and Umansky 1998), p.5)

Indeed, from an early-twentieth century Freudian conception of the mother as the first and central object of the infant's desires grew a mid-20th-century imperative for mothers to be omnipresent, unfailingly attentive and loving, and to derive deep satisfaction from that role. (Thurer 1993; Vicedo 2011) Alice Balint saw this imperative clearly in 1949, noting:

> The ideal mother has no interests of her own. ... For it remains self-evident that the interests of the mother and the child are identical, and it is the generally acknowledged measure of the goodness or badness of the mother how far she feels this identity of interests. (Balint 1949), p.252)

Even as mothers increasingly entered the workforce outside the home in the 1960s and 1970s, psychological attachment theorists continued to emphasize the importance of mothers who were ever-present without being overprotective, and who loved unselfishly without resentment. (Davis 1996); (Hays 1998); (Thurer 1993). Feminist scholars have for decades critiqued this "good mother" mandate as impossible to satisfy: "The institution of motherhood finds all mothers more or less guilty of having failed their children." (Rich 1995), p.223).

Today, as women gain increasing ability to monitor potential children earlier and earlier in pregnancy, the mandate to subsume herself to the interests of her child has merged with mandates for perfect bodily health (Williams et al. 2005) (Downing 2005) (Hallowell 1999; Steinberg 1996). In their theorization of "genetic responsibility," Carlos Novas and Nikolas Rose note that genetics now "operates in a political and ethical field in which individuals are increasingly obligated to formulate life strategies, to seek to maximize their life chances, to take actions or refrain from actions in order to increase the quality of their lives, and to act prudently in relation to themselves and to others." ((Novas and Rose 2000), p.487) These obligations figure prominently in social practices and discussions of health and health care policy as far back as the 1970s, when Robert Crawford observed the middle-class moralization of "healthism" emerging in response to rising healthcare costs and growing recognition of negative social and environmental health impacts. (Crawford 1980) This ethic, Crawford noted, "reinforces the privatization of the struggle for generalized well-being" (Crawford 1980), p.365) and "serves to reorder expectations and to justify a retreat from the language of rights and the policies of entitlements." ((Crawford 1977), p.668) Rather than expecting industry, government, and social institutions to provide more effectively for the health and welfare of workers and the general public, public policy and mass media have increasingly emphasized individual responsibility for health, and this ethic has been widely internalized, particularly among the middle class. More recently, Crawford has reflected, "individual responsibility for health has become a model of and a model for the neoliberal restructuring of American society." (Crawford 2006), pp. 419) In the reproductive sphere, the moral responsibility for individual health expands to include genetic responsibility for the future child. While women themselves may negotiate a complex calculus of responsibility to themselves, their partners and families, and their future child (Rapp 1999), social perspectives hold potential mothers "primarily accountable for the health of the fetus, and for making definitive decisions about prenatal testing and childbearing (Raspberry and Skinner 2011)." This rise of a middle-class ethic of individual responsibility for health and wellness (and for that of one's offspring) happened, not coincidentally, as an economic downturn began to threaten the security of the middle class in Western nations, and arguably has intensified as the middle class finds itself less economically secure, and more anxious about health, than ever.

8.3 Indirect Costs

In the midst of this trend, some economists began what would become an increasingly prevalent trend towards finding ways to not only glorify health, but quantify it. The concept of the indirect cost of illness or disability gained considerable favor in US health economics studies in the 1990s. Its roots lie in the post-WWII expansion of government agencies devoted to public safety and public health as an economic method of justifying government expenditure on regulation and health improvement. Considered objectively, for instance, the creation of an agency such as the Occupational Safety and Health Administration (OSHA) might be seen as a drain on taxpayer resources that also negatively affects business profits by requiring stricter safety standards and conducting regular inspections (Bartel and Thomas 1985; McCaffrey 2013). However, if one calculates the indirect costs of unsafe workplaces—the number of days off work, the number of workers' compensation claims for workplace-related accidents, the drain on public welfare systems from the families of individuals unable to work due to workplace accidents, the early retirement of workers due to accumulated disability in dangerous workplaces—it is clearer that the direct cost of creating regulation and enforcement to improve workplace safety may be outweighed by the cost, to the national economy as a whole, of lost productivity and increased burden on state-funded services (Rice et al. 1985; Rice 1967). This argument has been made to explain the systemic cost of a variety of conditions, including arthritis (Rat and Boissier 2004; Li et al. 2006) (Clarke et al. 1997), obesity and/or diabetes (Trogdon et al. 2008) (Colditz 1999) (Hoffman et al. 1996), and neurological conditions such as chronic migraines (Hu et al. 1999) and schizophrenia (Hu et al. 1996). As time went on, the 'indirect cost' of congenital conditions also began to be seen as an economic argument in favor of prenatal screening and testing. The cost of screening and termination, it was argued, would be offset by the money saved on medical support for the disabled and the loss of productive labor. (Benn et al. 2015).

While popular, and arguably effective, the concept of indirect cost is inherently flawed. One problem lies in its limitation to those conditions and individuals for which the only alternative activity—if the pathology in question were not present—would be full time paid employment. Tallying up the number of days workers did not attend work due to illness or estimating the burden of early retirement due to declining health does not accurately portray the impact of a health condition on society as a whole. These calculations do not take into account the flexibility of commercial enterprises to adjust to changes in workforce. Labor may be taken up by temporary workers, who would not otherwise be participating in the workforce, or by other employees through overtime work or extra shifts. If a worker retires early, the company is free to hire another worker, one who was previously unemployed (Koopmanschap et al. 1995). Thus, it is not clear that the indirect cost of a given health condition to the economy as a whole is as high as relatively primitive indirect cost measures would assume.

The second difficulty of indirect cost becomes clearer when the concept is expanded to more complex conditions such as diabetes, obesity, or mental illness. It is absolutely true that these conditions increase access to medical services, which may impact employer-provided health premiums, and may result in lost productivity or absence due to medical attendance or condition-related temporary disability. Certainly, these conditions may place considerable burden on individuals and their families, which is reason enough to support public health efforts towards their remediation. But as the medical establishment has been discovering for decades, these conditions are multifactorial, variable in severity, and highly contextualized. Calculating an 'indirect cost' that assumes that the only impact of such conditions is the number of otherwise economically productive days lost due to a medical condition is, to many, a dramatic oversimplification (Seuring, Archangelidi and Suhrcke 2015) (Cooper 2000) (Trogdon et al. 2008) (Jacobs and Fassbender, 1998).

A more conceptual point involves the way indirect costs are frequently framed as 'costs to society' rather than 'impact on GDP' or 'economic burden of disease.' Whether one uses a national approach—national loss of productive worker hours—or a household-specific one—loss of household income due to lost wages and medical costs—indirect costs can only accurately encompass impacts on a finite part of "social life": formalized paid employment by a designated corporate entity. A vast range of social and economic activity lies outside this realm, including unpaid household labor in childrearing and home maintenance; informal employment through art, music, freelance work, and undocumented work; philanthropy and other forms of public service; and the activities of individuals with fixed or pre-existing income, such as retirees or those with inherited wealth (Weinstein, Russell, Gold and Siegel 1996; Posnett and Jan 1996). As Jacobs and Fassbender point out, "Although the concepts of health-related quality of life and indirect costs are very closely related, they each measure different—but important—aspects of personal capabilities. The fact that such similar concepts appear in both the numerator and denominator [of cost effectiveness analyses] poses a dilemma for individuals who are trying to interpret cost-effectiveness results" (Jacobs and Fassbender, 1998).

8.4 Public Views on Prenatal Testing and the Cost of Disability

Perhaps more important than any of these debates, however, is the moral and ethical disjunction invoked by placing a monetary value on an individual's non-existence. One interesting phenomenon engendered by the rise of prenatal surveillance is the existence of so-called wrongful life suits: legal means by which an individual, or more commonly their parents, sue a medical provider for failing to inform them of a medical condition which might have led to elective pregnancy termination. The birth of a child with a disability is thus framed as a medical failure that must be economically redressed. While there have been rare instances of damages awarded in such cases, usually where malpractice can be relatively easily proven, most courts called to consider the issue have found that the benefit of being alive outweighs considerations of inadequacy in the quality of that life. (Sheth 2005) In the court of public opinion, however, judgments regarding which lives may not be worth living are inextricably entwined with the discourses of prenatal screening and testing.

In 2012 the Stanford Center for the Integration of Research on Genetics and Ethics fielded a custom website designed to solicit public engagement with emerging technologies. Using scenario building, an established tool of constructive technology assessment (Rip and Te Kulve, 2008), a team of multi-disciplinary experts—including genetic counselors, geneticists, sociologists, bioethicists, and maternal fetal medicine specialists—devised a scenario that depicted the clinical experience of a hypothetical 40-year-old patient named Cindy who was presented with four prenatal screening and testing options for fetal aneuploidy: no screening, a traditional (triple or quad) serum screen, prenatal screening using cell-free DNA (cfDNA), or amniocentesis. Actionability of screening results was presented as the ability either to make an informed choice about termination or to prepare for the birth of an affected child. The implicit and explicit narratives of disability that emerged from this study have been published previously (Steinbach, Allyse, Michie, Liu and Cho 2015). Below we explore some findings from this study that illustrate the intertwining of discourses of disability, health, cost, burden, responsibility, and motherhood within the arena of pregnancy and prenatal genetic testing.

More details about the methodology of this study are published elsewhere (Steinbach et al. 2015). Most relevant here is that the 220 participants who completed the online engagement exercise (ranging from 18 to 89 years old, and evenly split by gender) self-identified as coming from a wide variety of perspectives regarding prenatal screening and testing technologies, including parents, people who identified as disabled, medical professionals, special needs care providers and educators, and many who said they had no personal connection to these technologies. After answering a series of open-ended questions about their recommendations, participants were asked to read and respond to a series of alternative recommendations representing a range of perspectives (drawn from academic and public literature) that included examples from members of the disability community, parents of children with Down syndrome, and medical professionals. Below we include responses from various stages of the engagement scenario.

We found several distinct themes emerged that engaged with popular tropes surrounding health and productivity as markers of responsible motherhood and good citizenship. One was the belief that prenatal screening and testing, particularly under the circumstances of its availability in the US, illuminates existing injustice in the medico-technical system. In particular, respondents reacted to the fact that cfDNA screening was represented in the scenario as being more sensitive than traditional serum screening but at a much higher price point.

> This situation is much harder for people with no insurance, it is wrong that in the richest country in the world people should have to make these decisions with a system that wants to make money off of them and doesn't care very much for people that don't have money. [Male, 40]
>
> I believe every person has a right to an informed decision regardless of the expense. [Female, 43]

These respondents saw this injustice as unfairly targeting those of lower income and socioeconomic status, restricting access to tools that could allow families greater control over pregnancy decision-making and planning for the future health of their children. But other participants saw another kind of injustice resulting from restricting prenatal testing availability to those of greater financial resources: an injustice perpetrated on society in general.

> Unlike other countries where medical is provided, we must bear that burden. So if low income, where I'm sure a lot of Cindy's in our country come from, that's going to be more of a burden on taxpayers.... [T]here are two demographics here; ones that can afford, and those that can't. [Male, 43]

In this construct, the "burden" of disability resulting from continuing an affected pregnancy falls not on the family but on the social welfare system, as a result of a lack of subsidized health care and the limited resources of low income families. The injustice expressed here reflects both that low-income families do not have access to prenatal testing and that society must bear the "burden" of taking care of the disabled.

While within the themes above the lack of testing availability is portrayed as unjust, a separate theme expressed a contrasting view: that the availability of testing is an unjust judgment on the value of individuals with genetic conditions.

> She should have neither tests. Her baby has just as much chance to be born normal, or okay as any other baby… Any circumstance good or bad may be made joyous only by the way we look that baby in the eyes when they are born. Many Children grow to be outstanding people disability or not. [Female, 68]

From this perspective, treating an affected pregnancy differently than an unaffected one places unfair value on the calculus of health, without acknowledging the underlying intrinsic value of the child as a human being.

> I think the precautions with taking the tests are overboard. I am pro-life and believe that every child should be born despite their circumstances. It should be given a chance at least. I think some people give up too easy for what could be or what might happen. It is very selfish in my opinion for someone to abort a baby because it will affect their parents lifestyle. EVERY child does this regardless of a handicap or not. [Female, 36]

> It is a great thing technology but we are human not machine. We must live to our fullest. Sometimes the greatest things in our lives are the things we want least. [Male, 42]

Failure to give the affected pregnancy "a chance" is portrayed here as unjustly prioritizing the comfort and leisure of the parent over the rights of the fetus. This narrative reflects an implicit understanding of parents (specifically mothers, since the scenario exclusively addressed Cindy's decisions as a mother) as morally deficient if they are not willing to prioritize a future child's potential life over their own "lifestyle." Also implicit in this view is a form of virtue intrinsic to disability that enriches, rather than detracts from, family life.

This focus on the potential child as the rightful beneficiary of testing also emerged in a related theme that portrayed prenatal testing as supporting the rights of individuals to the healthiest future obtainable:

> [Not] all disabled children are born to loving parents, and those are the ones that must live an unhappy existence. The one thing I see is that people think about themselves and make a decision that makes them feel good. However, depending on the disability, no one makes the decision based on the quality of life the child will live… I believe the quality of life for a child is the top priority, and the effect a disabled child has on the entire family is just as important. I think it is less important how adults personally feel about their decision. [Female, 67]

Within this construct, the decision to undergo prenatal testing was again intimately linked to a willingness of a mother to subordinate her individual preferences to the well-being of the potential child. The decision not to undergo testing, or to select a less informative test over cfDNA screening, is here portrayed as a self-serving decision.

A very different, but even more explicit, description of selfishness emerged in other responses: the selfishness of allowing a disabled child to be born when prenatal screening could provide information that would justify elective termination.

> I think she should go with [cfDNA screening] only because the results [would] be more accurate and she would be able to make a better informed decision with the results afterwards. If the test comes back positive for DS, in my personal opinion, I would then opt to have a [sic] abortion. I do not believe that it is right to bring a child into the world knowing it is going to have a lifetime of difficulties ahead. I think it is selfish of the parent to bring it into the world just for the sake of satisfying their own conscience. [Male, 24]

> There is no justice in bringing in a disabled child into the world that can be prevented. It's not eugenics. It's a choice that affects whole families. It keeps the child from suffering throughout its entire life, never being able to integrate and live alone, saves the family from serious expenses, not to mention the potential loss of work from having to stay home at the kid. I find it irresponsible and even MORE harmful to the disabled child into this world, well knowing what the results and what their quality of life is going to be. [Male, 20]

While "difficulties" and "suffering" figured into these participants' imagination of life with a disability, a key component of this "justice" argument was the perceived inability of those with cognitive impairment to participate fully in society and to be productive rather than burdensome and costly. Refusing testing was thus portrayed by some respondents as a form of denying the potential future child full citizenship.

> Although the case can be made that many of those with Down syndrome are happy and lead fulfilling lives I can't help but think that this is a state of default unknown. They have never known anything more; so of course they can only understand they are "different" than others… Considering that I would personally look to abort the pregnancy…I think it's selfish in some capacity to have a child that is not able to take advantage of all life has to offer and is inherently at a disadvantage, regardless of whether or not the child was "happy" or not. [Male, 30]

Here, again, the decision to move forward with a pregnancy without the knowledge of future disability is characterized as "selfish," and potential parents are characterized as allowing their own desire to have a child (or to avoid the moral distress of contemplating abortion) to override the best interests of the potential child. In these responses runs a persistent current of belief that a less-than-healthy life is simply not worth living, and that choosing to prevent such a life is a more responsible form of motherhood than bringing it into the world.

An extension of the testing-as-justice theme is a portrayal of prenatal testing as a responsibility the potential parent owes not only to the potential child, but also to society at large. In this construct, the potentially disabled child negatively affects both its family and all of society.

> The only way I could see [cfDNA screening] affecting me would be if the cost of the child would some way become a burden on society. [Female, 56]

> Have the most reliable test [cfDNA screening]. If it's positive, she and her husband should seriously consider abortion… Kids are our most important resource, but a child who will not be self-sufficient is too much of a burden on society. [Male, 70]

This phrase, "burden on society," was repeated by several respondents, and was echoed by others who used similar wording to suggest that those with disabilities absorb a disproportionate share of social services and resources.

> No [cfDNA screening] [doesn't] affect me as far as children go, but it does affect me in the fact that I am a taxpayer and my taxes will pay for special schooling for this child, for possibly further health issues, and maybe financial support for the duration of its life. [Female, 58]

At their most extreme, responses in this theme suggested that prenatal testing was a form of civic duty. Such responses expanded the calculus of stakeholders in prenatal testing and/or termination decisions beyond the potential mother and her family into the larger social body of "taxpayers."

> If the test are [sic] positive one needs to know if they can handle what lies before them in their future. This is where they need to decide to end the pregnancy or raise the child the best possible realizing that this will be a forever job. It will not end at 18 years old like a normal child. Can they live with this? If not, I believe they should end the pregnancy unless they know someone who wants to take the responsibility and raise that child to be happy as possible and not raise them to get money from the state... This may seem callous but why should the state pay for our mistakes as parents, and breeding without regard to health issues. Just because we can reproduce does not mean we should… [Female, 48]

Notably, this view did not necessitate recommending abortion of affected pregnancies. Rather, respondents expressed that the responsibility of the potential parent was to consider whether they had sufficient resources to raise an affected child on their own. Again, the decision to move forward with a pregnancy without the knowledge of future disability is characterized as "selfish"; and potential parents are characterized as allowing their desire to avoid the moral distress of contemplating abortion to override the best interests of the potential child.

8.5 Pathways to Affluence

The findings from this study reflect a consciousness of the larger social narratives we have described above: that individual health and the economics of both family and society are intimately connected and that, to many, the imperative to be responsible for having "healthy" children (that do not "burden" family and society) should override any other aspect of motherhood. Mothers are now expected to be "good" long before their children are even born, and in ways that extend well beyond emotional availability and basic physical needs. The science of reproduction has progressed to include ever more accurate and accessible prenatal screening and testing technologies; and women's decisions about whether and how to use these, and what to do with the information from them, take place in dialogue both with notions of good mothering and with neoliberal discourses of responsibility for individual bodies and health.

In social discourses of the good mother and of individual responsibility for health, social and economic security are both implicit precursors and implicitly protected. In order to be a good (pregnant) mother, a woman must have the means to do so; and in taking appropriate responsibility for the health of her future children, she also protects the socioeconomic future of her family. In her interviews with pregnant women, Deborah Lupton found—particularly among middle-class women—a hyper-awareness of fetal risks and vigilance regarding their own behavior. She suggested, "For middle-class women, in particular, this opportunity to attempt to reassert control over the uncertainty and unruliness of pregnancy may be welcome, conforming as it does to bourgeois ideals of autonomy, self-control and the care of the self." (Lupton 2012), p.332) Dorothy Roberts (Roberts 2009) notes that such discourses and practices are classed, raced, and gendered. While largely privatized infertility services are less accessible to poor and minority populations, prenatal screening and testing are often subsidized by public insurance. And as the focus of self-regulation in the context of reproductive genetics and fetal risk, "women bear the brunt of reprogenetics' contribution to the neoliberal restructuring of health care." ((Roberts 2009), p.794) In this context of individualized genetic responsibility, middle class women know that the "choice" not to test for fetal genetic conditions—or to continue a pregnancy diagnosed with them—likely entails giving up an already shaky hold on economic security for both themselves and their children, while poor and marginalized women know that this "choice" likely means giving up on dreams of gaining such security. Such a context makes "choice" a misnomer, as Abby Lippman argues: "If prenatal testing and abortion of fetuses with the disability constitute the only solution offered, a need for screening gets created." ((Lippman 1991), p.20).

As these economic, social, and technological trends historically converged in the last third of the twentieth century, prenatal screening and testing quickly took on the cloak of responsible motherhood, as the role of good mothers began incorporating responsible use of genetic technologies during pregnancy to "not only assure but also insure their baby's health." ((Press and Browner 1993), p.105) Remarking in the early 1990s on the "speed and completeness of its acceptance," Lisa Ikemoto observed, "Amniocentesis may seem so obviously beneficial, and so low risk, that using it as an example [of the regulation of pregnant women] appears inappropriate or paranoid." (Ikemoto 1992), p.1291) In comparison, today's prenatal cfDNA screening, lacking even the small iatrogenic risks of amniocentesis, has found acceptance among both patients and providers at a speed that is "unprecedented in the history of prenatal care." ((Chitty and Bianchi 2013), p.511).

8.6 Profiting From the Pathway

Unlike previous prenatal screening and testing technologies, prenatal cfDNA screening has not grown up within the relatively controlled confines of hospitals and public health programs. The technology necessary to isolate and sequence placental DNA in maternal serum was patented very shortly after its discovery and publication by Dennis Lo in 1997 (Lo et al. 1997). Subsequent methods have also been patented and commercialized, with the result that by 2019, industry giants such as Illumina, Roche, and BGI owned and invested heavily in intellectual property around prenatal sequencing. However, these highly successful economic actors would not invest heavily in a technology unless they predicted significant return on investment. The goal of investing in pharmaceuticals, for instance, is to find a drug that successfully ameliorates a disease state and to profit from selling it back to the health care system. In this case, profit from prenatal cfDNA screens is dependent upon clinicians offering, and women accepting, prenatal genetic screening. Indeed, many industry-linked cost effectiveness studies assume universal global uptake of genetic screening during pregnancy (Song, Musci and Caughey 2013).

The problems with this assumption, however, are two-fold: historically not all women have had access to prenatal screening, and many of those who are offered various forms of such screening decline it (Kuppermann et al. 2006) (Sayres et al. 2014). Past studies have shown that women with inconsistent access to health care are less likely to present for prenatal care (or they present later in pregnancy) (Phillippi 2009; Ruwe et al. 2010; Bryant et al. 2010); and women from some ethnic groups, including Hispanic and Black (Kuppermann et al. 1996), and some religious groups, in particular Catholic and some evangelical faiths (Sayres et al. 2014), are more likely to decline screening and testing. Although the numbers disguise considerable variation by geographical region and urban/rural divides, on average between 67 and 72% of women in the US have historically undergone prenatal screening (Palomaki et al. 2013). This number is even lower in some European countries, despite the availability of universal healthcare (Crombag et al. 2014; Loane et al. 2013; Rowe, Garcia and Davidson 2004; Boyd et al. 2008). And in low- and middle-income nations with high population growth, including India, decentralized health systems make it difficult to assess how many women are receiving formal medical care during pregnancy at all, let alone genetic screening (Mozersky et al. 2017; Chandrasekharan et al. 2014; Verma et al. 2012; Kaur et al. 2012). The other challenge for cfDNA is that many areas already have prenatal screening systems in place. Serum marker screening is cheap, well integrated into public health systems, and widely understood and interpreted by prenatal providers. This landscape has presented companies with a potentially formidable challenge: how to convince more women and healthcare payor entities that prenatal *genetic* screening is absolutely essential and should be universally adopted?

Companies have responded by investing heavily in marketing and political strategy. One key approach has been to build tests that reflect and dovetail with familiar screening programs and conditions. The focus has been on integrating the new technology into existing regulatory and clinical pathways as an established health care need that has merely been improved by the introduction of genetics. It is no accident that the first commercially available cfDNA screen in the US was designed to detect only one condition: Down syndrome. Down syndrome is the keystone of prenatal screening and testing, the single genetic condition parents are most familiar with and the centerpiece of counseling and education on prenatal screening and diagnosis. The relative ease of detecting Down syndrome with cfDNA, while certainly a factor in choosing the initial focus of this screening technology, may have carried less weight than the simple fact that Down syndrome is the condition (often the only genetic condition) that most pregnant mothers are aware of when they walk into their first prenatal clinic visit. Following this familiar social pathway (Callon 1986) and exceeding previous expectations of existing non-invasive screens (serum screening and ultrasound), prenatal cfDNA laboratories have both expanded panels to include many more conditions and also pushed more and more aggressively for expanded access to all pregnancies. Indeed, companies have begun aggressive political lobbying for Medicaid coverage of prenatal cfDNA screens in all pregnancies (see, for example, the industry-created website capsprenatal.com)—couching this lobbying in the language of "health disparities," but focusing exclusively on their commercial product rather than the basic pregnancy services that many Medicaid plans fail to provide to women.

A second key strategy has been to market tests using the familiar tropes of health, responsibility, and affluence. Marketing materials typically show happy, healthy pregnant couples surrounded by subtle markers of affluence such as uncluttered, all-white living areas, or unencumbered access to pristine natural settings. The language of marketing materials directed at patients echoes themes of responsibility and reassurance. "It's natural to have concerns about the health of your unborn baby," one pamphlet affirmed, adding, "But prenatal testing can help reduce these concerns." Words like "reassured" and the phrase "peace of mind" pop up often in these materials, suggesting that a pregnancy with screen-negative cfDNA results allows mothers to let go of "natural" anxieties that they have not fulfilled their duty to produce a healthy child. These assurances sit alongside language of consumer empowerment: "It's your pregnancy," marketers say, with imperatives to "demand" the "accuracy" or "clarity" of their brand of test. "Empower yourself," they repeat over and over: "Your baby deserves the best." While tropes equating knowledge with power and encouraging good consumerism to "demand the best" are commonplace in advertising, in the setting of an optional screening test for a future child's genetic conditions, these tropes connect implicitly to deep cultural imperatives of responsible motherhood. When you are a responsible mother, your baby deserves the best that you can give her, whatever the cost to you—and anything less is deficient mothering. Little wonder, then, that the language of responsibility (and its antithesis, "selfishness") has cropped up so often in our research. As a woman we interviewed in 2013 described her decision to have prenatal cfDNA screening, "I wanted to do my due diligence, especially because there was no risk. … It's about the well-being of the child. It's being responsible for the child's health and thinking about what I could do." The phrase "due diligence," with its overt connections to legal obligations and business contracts, enlarged this mother's sense of responsibility into a metaphorical contractual obligation, arguably not only with her potential child but with the social future that child engendered. It is this implicit and burdensome sense of maternal responsibility that companies know they tap into with their marketing images and language of "empowerment" and "reassurance."

A third key strategy has been to frame prenatal cfDNA screening as a cost savings measure designed to reduce the burden on the health system. Here, again, the focus has been on Down syndrome as not only the most widely recognized trisomy but also the most compatible with relatively long lifespan. Employees of testing companies and academics with whom they have a financial relationship have repeatedly argued that prenatal cfDNA screening should be offered as a first-tier screen to all expectant women because universal cfDNA screening would allow for identification of more pregnancies affected by Down syndrome and reduction in the "cost of care of Down syndrome, which we all know is significant" (Fairbrother et al. 2015).

This line of argument, in discussions of disabling conditions, is hardly new. In a 1976 BMJ article, Hagard and Spencer reported that "prevention" of Down syndrome live births as a result of diagnosis via amniocentesis could result in "economic benefits" of UK£805,587. They noted, however: "[O]ur conclusions rest on the assumption that those responsible for health planning embrace the cost–benefit analysis approach, *perceiving their responsibilities beyond the narrow framework of health services*" [emphasis added] (Hagard and Carter 1976) In their 2005 analysis, Odibo et al. reported that restructuring screening strategies would "result in… a societal savings of $8,516 per additional [Down syndrome] case averted". (Odibo et al. 2005). In their 2015 analysis, Benn et al. assessed the "lifetime cost" of Down syndrome at between US$541,600–812,400 and argued that "replacing conventional screening with NIPT [cfDNA] would increase fetal aneuploidy detection rates, decrease the number of affected births, and lower the number of invasive tests and thereby reduce procedure-related losses of euploid fetuses." (Benn et al. 2015) Notably, the model conceded that prenatal cfDNA screening was significantly more expensive than existing public health screens, but maintained that these costs would be offset by societal savings from the termination of pregnancies affected by Down syndrome rather than long-term care of the children that might result. (Benn et al. 2015) The "cost-effectiveness" argument is that all women should be receiving cfDNA screening in order to avoid the "price for the birth of a child affected with one of the trisomies" (Karow 2015), and its implication is that all women should accept prenatal screening and testing in order to save themselves, and the rest of society, the burden of individuals with special needs. These arguments closely echo those in our study's scenario responses that suggest women, in making decisions about continuing a pregnancy, have an obligation not only to consider the financial needs of their family but also to be ready to sacrifice the pregnancy if necessary for the wider good of society. Prenatal genetic testing is the tool that allows mothers to know whether that sacrifice is necessary.

8.7 Beyond Down Syndrome

> "Technological advancement and several benefits associated with infant genetic testing will be major driver of the prenatal and newborn genetic testing market. Introduction of prenatal testing has led to substantial amount of increase in adoption rate of new testing technologies

> such as non-invasive prenatal testing (NIPT) for detection of sub chromosomal abnormalities, single-gene disorders and aneuploidy in North America region. Inclination towards minimally invasive infant genetic testing along with demand for early detection of birth defects will one of the major reason for market growth."[1]

As commercial cfDNA laboratories eye ever-larger markets for their screening tests, they will need to continue making a strong argument that fetal genetic conditions pose a threat to individual health, family well-being, and social welfare. This argument has already proven effective regarding Down syndrome and other common aneuploidies, especially among middle- and upper-class women in high-income nations. And legitimate public health arguments can be made for prenatal screening for certain conditions, especially in certain populations. Thalessemia disorders, for instance, are acknowledged as a heavy public health burden in the Middle East and parts of east Asia, suggesting that a prenatal screen that could effectively identify these conditions earlier in pregnancy would be very attractive to health officials and many families. It is not clear, however, that the wholesale expansion of prenatal genetic screening is targeted to the legitimate public health needs of society, rather than simply creating more reasons why women need these tests. Most of the largest prenatal cfDNA screening companies in 2019 offer a panel of microdeletion conditions—some of which are so rare that actual incidence cannot be determined—and for all of these, cfDNA screening offers positive predictive values below 25%. In removing prenatal screening from the healthcare realm and situating it in the commercial one, we have apparently severed the connection that ideally ties the intervention (screening) to the goal of the intervention (clinical utility and care).

Nevertheless, the push continues, not only for more numerous and varied fetal conditions, but also among a broader population that may be less convinced by the image of the technologically-empowered, economically stable, and socially responsible "good mother." As screening panels grow, the image of the future "healthy" child narrows, and the conditions for which "responsible" mothers should be vigilant become increasingly less familiar and more unlikely. Yet as target populations broaden, mothers' own goals for their children and images of ideal families are necessarily more and more diverse. The argument that mothers should choose the most cutting-edge test, offering the most accuracy regarding the greatest number of conditions, will likely continue in force, but its specifics are likely to be increasingly vague: stripped down to its barest essence, the claim is simply that potential mothers carry the heavy weight of responsibility for their future child's every possibility.

---

[1] https://www.openpr.com/news/1696401/What-s-driving-the-Prenatal-and-New-born-Genetic-Testing-market-Share-Ariosa-Diagnostics-Roche-Berry-Genomics-BGI-Biorad-Illumina-Laboratory-Corporation-of-America-Natera-Qiagen-Sequenom-Trivitron-Healthcare-and-Verinata-health.html

References

Balint, M. 1949. Early developmental states of the ego. Primary object love. *International Journal of Psycho-Analysis* 30: 265–273.

Bartel, A.P., and L.G. Thomas. 1985. Direct and indirect effects of regulation: A new look at OSHA's impact. *The Journal of Law and Economics* 28 (1): 1–25.

Benn, P., Curnow, K. J., Chapman, S., Michalopoulos, S. N., Hornberger, J., and M. Rabinowitz. 2015. An economic analysis of cell-free DNA non-invasive prenatal testing in the US General pregnancy population. *PLoS One* 10(7): e0132313.

Boyd, P. A., DeVigan, C., Khoshnood, B., Loane, M., Garne, E., Dolk, H., and EUROCAT Working Group. (2008). Survey of prenatal screening policies in Europe for structural malformations and chromosome anomalies, and their impact on detection and termination rates for neural tube defects and Down's syndrome. *BJOG: An International Journal of Obstetrics & Gynaecology* 115(6): 689–696.

Bryant, A.S., A. Worjoloh, A.B. Caughey, and A.E. Washington. 2010. Racial/ethnic disparities in obstetric outcomes and care: Prevalence and determinants. *American Journal of Obstetrics and Gynecology* 202 (4): 335–343.

Callon, M. 1986. The sociology of an actor-network: The case of the electric vehicle. In *Mapping the dynamics of science and technology* (pp. 19–34). London, Palgrave McMillan.

Chandrasekharan, S., Minear, M. A., Hung, A., and M. Allyse. 2014. Noninvasive prenatal testing goes global. *Science Translational Medicine* 6(231): 231fs15–231fs15.

Chitty, L.S., and D.W. Bianchi. 2013. Noninvasive prenatal testing: The paradigm is shifting rapidly. *Prenatal Diagnosis* 33 (6): 511–513.

Clarke, A.E., H. Zowall, C. Levinton, H. Assimakopoulos, J.T. Sibley, M. Haga, and S.A. Grover. 1997. Direct and indirect medical costs incurred by Canadian patients with rheumatoid arthritis: A 12 year study. *The Journal of Rheumatology* 24 (6): 1051–1060.

Colditz, G.A. 1999. Economic costs of obesity and inactivity. *Medicine and Science in Sports and Exercise* 31 (11 Suppl): S663–S667.

Cooper, N.J. 2000. Economic burden of rheumatoid arthritis: A systematic review. *Rheumatology* 39 (1): 28–33.

Crawford, R. 1977. You are dangerous to your health: The ideology and politics of victim blaming. *International Journal of Health Services* 7 (4): 663–680.

Crawford, R. 1980. Healthism and the medicalization of everyday life. *International Journal of Health Services* 10 (3): 365–388.

Crawford, R. 2006. Health as a meaningful social practice. *Health* 10 (4): 401–420.

Crombag, N.M.T.H., Y.E. Vellinga, S.A. Kluijfhout, L.D. Bryant, P.A. Ward, R. Iedema-Kuiper, and A. Tabor. 2014. Explaining variation in Down's syndrome screening uptake: Comparing the Netherlands with England and Denmark using documentary analysis and expert stakeholder interviews. *BMC Health Services Research* 14 (1): 437.

Davis, P.C. 1996. The good mother: A new look at psychological parent theory. *NYU Rev. L. & Soc. Change* 22: 347.

Downing, C. 2005. Negotiating responsibility: Case studies of reproductive decision-making and prenatal genetic testing in families facing Huntington disease. *Journal of Genetic Counseling* 14 (3): 219–234.

Fairbrother, G., Burigo, J., Sharon, T., and K. Song. 2015. Prenatal screening for fetal aneuploidies with cell-free DNA in the general pregnancy population: a cost-effectiveness analysis. *The Journal of Maternal-Fetal & Neonatal Medicine*: 1–5.

Hagard, S., and F.A. Carter. 1976. Preventing the birth of infants with Down's syndrome: A cost-benefit analysis. *BMJ* 1 (6012): 753–756.

Hallowell, N. 1999. Doing the right thing: Genetic risk and responsibility. *Sociology of Health & Illness* 21 (5): 597–621.

Hays, S. 1998. *The cultural contradictions of motherhood*. New Haven, Yale University Press.

Hoffman, C., D. Rice, and H.-Y. Sung. 1996. Persons with chronic conditions: Their prevalence and costs. *JAMA* 276 (18): 1473–1479.

Hu, T.-W., Hargreaves, W. A., and M. Shumway. 1996. Estimating costs of schizophrenia and its treatment. In *Handbook of mental health economics and health policy. Handbook of mental health economics and health policy, Vol. 1*. M. Moscarelli, A. R., & N. Sartorius (Eds.), *Schizophrenia*, 359–371. Oxford, England: John Wiley & Sons.

Hu, X.H., L.E. Markson, R.B. Lipton, W.F. Stewart, and M.L. Berger. 1999. Burden of migraine in the United States: Disability and economic costs. *Archives of Internal Medicine* 159 (8): 813–818.

Ikemoto, L.C. 1992. The code of perfect pregnancy: At the intersection of the ideology of motherhood, the practice of defaulting to science, and the interventionist mindset of law. *Ohio St. LJ* 53: 1205.

Jacobs, P., and K. Fassbender. 1998. The measurement of indirect costs in the health economics evaluation literature: A review. *International Journal of Technology Assessment in Health Care* 14 (4): 799–808.

Karow, L. 2015. NIPT Outperforms Standard Screening for T21 but False Positives Call for Caution, NEJM Studies Find. *Genomeweb*. NIPT Outperforms Standard Screening for T21 but False Positives Call for Caution, NEJM Studies Find. https://www.genomeweb.com/reproductive-health/nipt-outperforms-standard-screening-t21-false-positives-call-caution-nejm. Accessed Nov 7 2021.

Kaur, G., J. Srivastav, A. Kaur, A. Huria, P. Goel, R. Kaur, and P. Aggarwal. 2012. Maternal serum second trimester screening for chromosomal disorders and neural tube defects in a government hospital of North India. *Prenatal Diagnosis* 32 (12): 1192–1196.

Koopmanschap, M.A., F.F.H. Rutten, B.M. van Ineveld, and L. Van Roijen. 1995. The friction cost method for measuring indirect costs of disease. *Journal of Health Economics* 14 (2): 171–189.

Kuppermann, M., E. Gates, and A. E. Washington. 1996. Racial-ethnic differences in prenatal diagnostic test use and outcomes: Preferences, socioeconomics, or patient knowledge? *Obstetrics & Gynecology* 87 (5): 675–682.

Kuppermann, M., L.A. Learman, E. Gates, S.E. Gregorich, R.F. Nease Jr., J. Lewis, and A.E. Washington. 2006. Beyond race or ethnicity and socioeconomic status: Predictors of prenatal testing for Down syndrome. *Obstetrics & Gynecology* 107 (5): 1087.

Ladd-Taylor, M., and L. Umansky. 1998. *"Bad" mothers: The politics of blame in twentieth-century America*. New York, New York: NYU Press.

Li, X., Gignac, M. A. M., and A.H. Anis. 2006. The indirect costs of arthritis resulting from unemployment, reduced performance, and occupational changes while at work. *Medical care* 44 (4): 304–310.

Lippman, A. 1991. Prenatal genetic testing and screening: Constructing needs and reinforcing inequities. *Am. JL & Med.* 17: 15.

Lo, Y. M., Corbetta, N., Chamberlain, P. F., Rai, V., Sargent, I. L., Redman, C. W. G., and J. S. Wainscoat. 1997. Presence of fetal DNA in maternal plasma and serum. *The Lancet* 350(9076): 485–487.

Loane, M., J.K. Morris, M.-C. Addor, L. Arriola, J. Budd, B. Doray, and B. Khoshnood. 2013. Twenty-year trends in the prevalence of Down syndrome and other trisomies in Europe: Impact of maternal age and prenatal screening. *European Journal of Human Genetics* 21 (1): 27.

Lupton, D. 2012. 'Precious cargo': Foetal subjects, risk and reproductive citizenship. *Critical Public Health* 22 (3): 329–340.

McCaffrey, D. P. 2013. *OSHA and the Politics of Health Regulation*. Springer Science & Business Media.

Mozersky, J., V. Ravitsky, R. Rapp, M. Michie, S. Chandrasekharan, and M. Allyse. 2017. Toward an ethically sensitive implementation of noninvasive prenatal screening in the global context. *Hastings Center Report* 47 (2): 41–49.

Novas, C., and N. Rose. 2000. Genetic risk and the birth of the somatic individual. *Economy and Society* 29 (4): 485–513.

Odibo, A.O., D.M. Stamilio, D.B. Nelson, H.M. Sehdev, and G.A. Macones. 2005. A cost-effectiveness analysis of prenatal screening strategies for Down syndrome. *Obstetrics & Gynecology* 106 (3): 562–568.

Palomaki, G.E., G.J. Knight, E.R. Ashwood, R.G. Best, and J.E. Haddow. 2013. Screening for Down syndrome in the United States: Results of surveys in 2011 and 2012. *Archives of Pathology and Laboratory Medicine* 137 (7): 921–926.

Phillippi, J.C. 2009. Women's perceptions of access to prenatal care in the United States: A literature review. *Journal of Midwifery & Women's Health* 54 (3): 219–225.

Posnett, J., and S. Jan. 1996. Indirect cost in economic evaluation: The opportunity cost of unpaid inputs. *Health Economics* 5 (1): 13–23.

Press, N.A., and C.H. Browner. 1993. 'Collective fictions': Similarities in reasons for accepting maternal serum alpha-fetoprotein screening among women of diverse ethnic and social class backgrounds. *Fetal Diagnosis and Therapy* 8 (Suppl. 1): 97–106.

Rapp, R. 1999. *Testing women, testing the fetus: The social impact of amniocentesis in America New York*, New York: Routledge.

Raspberry, K., and D. Skinner. 2011. Enacting genetic responsibility: Experiences of mothers who carry the fragile X gene. *Sociology of Health & Illness* 33 (3): 420–433.

Rat, A.-C., and M.-C. Boissier. 2004. Rheumatoid arthritis: Direct and indirect costs. *Joint, Bone, Spine* 71 (6): 518–524.

Rice, D.P. 1967. Estimating the cost of illness. *American Journal of Public Health and the Nations Health* 57 (3): 424–440.

Rice, D.P., T.A. Hodgson, and A.N. Kopstein. 1985. The economic costs of illness: A replication and update. *Health Care Financing Review* 7 (1): 61.

Rich, A. 1995. *Of woman born: Motherhood as experience and institution*. WW Norton & Company.

Rip A., Kulve H. (2008) Constructive Technology Assessment and Socio-Technical Scenarios. In: Fisher E., Selin C., Wetmore J.M. (eds) *Presenting Futures. The Yearbook of Nanotechnology in Society, vol 1*. Dordrecht: Springer.

Roberts, D. E. 2009. Race, gender, and genetic technologies: A new reproductive dystopia. *Signs: Journal of Women in Culture and Society* 34(4): 783–804.

Rowe, R.E., J. Garcia, and L.L. Davidson. 2004. Social and ethnic inequalities in the offer and uptake of prenatal screening and diagnosis in the UK: A systematic review. *Public Health* 118 (3): 177–189.

Ruwe, M., J. Capitman, M. Bengiamin, and T. Soto. 2010. A systematic review and meta-analysis of racial disparities in prenatal care in California: How much? Does insurance matter. *Social Work in Public Health* 25 (6): 550–571.

Sayres, L. C., Allyse, M., Goodspeed, T. A., and M. K. Cho. 2014. Demographic and experiential correlates of public attitudes towards cell-free fetal DNA screening. *Journal of Genetic Counseling* 23 (6): 957–967.

Seuring, T., O. Archangelidi, and M. Suhrcke. 2015. The economic costs of type 2 diabetes: A global systematic review. *PharmacoEconomics* 33 (8): 811–831.

Sheth, D.M. 2005. Better off unborn? An analysis of wrongful birth and wrongful life claims under the Americans with Disabilities Act. *Tenn. L. Rev.* 73: 641.

Song, K., T.J. Musci, and A.B. Caughey. 2013. Clinical utility and cost of non-invasive prenatal testing with cfDNA analysis in high-risk women based on a US population. *The Journal of Maternal-Fetal & Neonatal Medicine* 26 (12): 1180–1185.

Steinbach, R. J., Allyse, M., Michie, M., Liu, E. Y., and M. K. Cho. 2015. "This lifetime commitment": Public conceptions of disability and noninvasive prenatal genetic screening. *American Journal of Medical Genetics* 170(2): 363–374.

Steinberg, D. L. (1996). Languages of risk: genetic encryptions of the female body. *Women: A Cultural Review* 7(3): 259–270.

Thurer, S. 1993. Changing conceptions of the good mother in psychoanalysis. *Psychoanalytic Review* 80 (4): 519–540.

Trogdon, J.G., E.A. Finkelstein, T. Hylands, P.S. Dellea, and S.J. Kamal-Bahl. 2008. Indirect costs of obesity: A review of the current literature. *Obesity Reviews* 9 (5): 489–500.
Verma, I.C., M. Lall, and R.D. Puri. 2012. Down syndrome in India—Diagnosis, screening, and prenatal diagnosis. *Clinics in Laboratory Medicine* 32 (2): 231–248.
Vicedo, M. 2011. The social nature of the mother's tie to her child: John Bowlby's theory of attachment in post-war America. *The British Journal for the History of Science* 44 (3): 401–426.
Weinstein, M.C., L.B. Russell, M.R. Gold, and J.E. Siegel. 1996. *Cost-effectiveness in health and medicine*. Oxford, England: Oxford University Press.
Williams, C., J. Sandall, G. Lewando-Hundt, B. Heyman, K. Spencer, and R. Grellier. 2005. Women as moral pioneers? Experiences of first trimester antenatal screening. *Social Science & Medicine* 61 (9): 1983–1992.

Part IV
The Future?

Chapter 9
An Intelligent Parents Guide to Prenatal Testing: Having a Well-Born Child Without Genomic Selection

David Wasserman

Abstract This imaginative guide to decision-making about prenatal genomics is situated in a not-too-distant future in which parents can easily choose among embryos from gametes that have been produced in a laboratory using their own skin cells. Readers are invited into a future vision of conscientious parenting that involves testing to protect, rather than to select, a future child.

So you're planning to have a child? You've just discovered that your insurance will pay for PSEDIVG. In case you haven't been following the science news, that's Preimplantation Selection of Embryos Derived from In Vitro Gametogenesis. It lets you and your partner create an array of embryos from gametes produced in a laboratory from your skin cells. Those embryos undergo PGD (surely you know that one!—Preimplantation Genetic Diagnosis) using WGS (and that! —Whole Genome Sequencing). You can learn everything that can be genetically ascertained or predicted about the kind of child that will develop from each embryo—and these days, that's quite a lot. You can even specify the conditions and traits for which you get test results. There's a small catch: the insurer won't pay unless you agree not to implant an embryo with genetic features predisposing it to any condition on a fairly short list of Very Serious Diseases and Disabilities (VSDDs). Aside from that, you're free to pick whichever embryo you want, by whatever criteria you choose.

So why are we advising you to think twice about this incredible freebie? Are we Luddites or (worse) Bioconservatives? Hardly. We love genomic technology, we promote the judicious use of prenatal genetic therapy, and we don't lose sleep over the boundaries between therapy and enhancement. We are almost scandalously nonchalant about the threat to humanity posed by posthuman carnivores, evil mutant geniuses, and superbugs, let alone by overpopulation or global warming. But we do worry that the new selection technologies will give you options you may regret

D. Wasserman (✉)
Department of Bioethics, NIH Clinical Center, College Park, USA
e-mail: david.wasserman@nih.gov

University of Maryland, College Park, MD 20742, USA

M. A. Allyse and M. Michie (eds.), *Born Well: Prenatal Genetics and the Future of Having Children*, The International Library of Bioethics 88,
https://doi.org/10.1007/978-3-030-82536-2_9

having and encourage you to make choices that you probably should decline to make. We urge you to resist a siren song that will lure you into an anxious, oppressive perfectionism. Here are some tips for binding yourself to the mast.

9.1 Too Much Information, Too Many Choices

(1) You've got an almost endless number of skin cells to spare, and it costs the lab only cents to convert a pair into an embryo. It's only a few cents more to do WGS on each of the ones you produce. There's an embryo limit—check your policy for specifics—but it's typically in the double digits, maybe triple. So you can get a lot of information on a lot of embryos. We hope you like digesting reams of data and making tough choices! Remember, you get to implant only one embryo. Did we forget to mention that your insurance policy will only cover 2 hours of genetic counseling? That might be fine if you had only one, maybe two, embryos to consider. But with an array of any size, you're going to be on your own after getting some pretty generic advice. Even if you're lucky enough to have a platinum policy with two or three times the counseling hours, no amount of counseling is going to be much help in dealing with all the probabilities of all the traits and conditions that you'll be receiving. Certainly, you don't want an embryo that's unlikely to survive gestation, or a child unlikely to survive more than a few months or years. Maybe you don't want a child with a high probability of a VSDD (We'll get to that later). But beyond that?

Every one of those ever-so-many embryos is going to have a not-insignificant probability of developing some nasty condition or trait. Almost every one of those embryos is going to have a not-insignificant probability of developing, at least with your investment, some traits that you would cherish as parents. Almost every one, except the small fraction you can screen out as likely to have totally awful lives, represents a complex package of possible traits and vulnerabilities. Even if you didn't have to worry about probabilities, with so many combinations and so many ways of living well (and badly), how would you decide whether one combination was better than another, let alone which one was the best?

(2) Maybe you think you could preserve your sanity by doing what economists call "satisficing" —settling for "good enough" when "better" is speculative, debatable, or not all that important. Maybe you could take one embryo at a time: once you got one whose results were "good enough," you'd just implant it. Satisficing *might* work, if you had high tolerance for risk and a lot of discipline and self-restraint. You'd need a high tolerance for risk because you could hardly be sure whether the child who would develop from that embryo would actually have a good enough life. Maybe you should hold out for one with an even higher probability of doing at least OK. You'd need discipline and self-restraint because you could keep on looking for just pennies more. Maybe the next embryo you tested would have even better odds of an even better package of traits, and even lower odds of the kinds of disease and disability you worry about. It may be incredibly hard to stop; if you're tempted to continue, you're likely to decide that the embryo you just tested wasn't really "good enough" after all.

(3) Maybe you think you could draw a sharp line to limit your choices by testing only for VSDDs from a small batch of embryos. You could certainly do that, as long as you were willing to accept your insurer's judgment about what conditions were so bad to be worth selecting against. But why should you? It's a list is based on the estimated health care costs of those conditions, which your insurer would have to cover unless it specifically excluded them. Maybe you *should* take those costs into account (again, we'll discuss this later), but not for your insurer's sake. And you'll be concerned about so much more than healthcare costs.

In general, you'll likely find your insurer's official VSDD list ill-suited to guide your own deliberations. On the one hand, you may find it underinclusive. It probably doesn't include genetic variants that predispose to mild cognitive impairment or chronic pain, for example, unless those variants also increase health care costs. Cognitive impairment or chronic pain alone won't cost health insurers much, but you may be reluctant to raise a child such conditions (once again, see below). On the other hand, you may find the list over-inclusive. What if an embryo with a VSDD also had the genetic potential for great intellectual or artistic achievements? Think about Stephen Hawking, the famous astrophysicist who had ALS—the disease that bears his name (for you old-timers, it used to be named for Lou Gehrig—whoever he was.) Several genetic variants have now been identified predisposing to that condition, and they're on the list. Rather than reject a potential genius, you might be tempted to test for positive traits as well—which we can now do to a limited extent. And if you're testing for those traits in some embryos, why not in all of them?

(4) Of course, there's only so much you can learn from the test results. Selecting on the basis of genetic features remains a game of chance. Even with the powerful diagnostic and predictive technologies we now possess, the outcome is still a crapshoot. The kind of child you have, and how its life goes, will be largely determined by external circumstances and events. Certainly, you can improve the odds of certain outcomes by genetic selection (e.g. *against* specific diseases, *for* height, pitch, or certain intellectual and athletic abilities), but much of the variation in most of the outcomes you care about isn't attributable to genetic features.

Most of the bad (and good) things that will happen to your children cannot be predicted from their genes, now or ever. Many more disabilities are caused by injuries and disease—injuries and disease to which "all flesh is heir," not just some genetically predisposed minority. You can certainly improve the odds that you will have a child who will outlive you by selecting against specific, and fairly rare, genetic conditions. You can reduce the odds of having a child who will die of certain cancers or cardiovascular diseases. But the apparently able-bodied future children you end up selecting may die young from a communicable disease, a street crime, a war (of choice or necessity), a drug overdose, a household accident, or a car crash. The number of children who will die from such (almost) entirely nongenomic causes is vastly greater than the number of future children who would die of genetic diseases (if they were not excluded prenatally). So unless you have a family history than gives your next child a 25% or 50% chance of having a deadly condition, the overall risk reduction from prenatal selection is pretty negligible. But apart from premature death, which is becoming increasingly rare in the second quarter of the twenty-first century, your child may be unlucky in love, friendship, or work; bodily harms are only one source of human misery, and far from the most important. Some people respond that since life is so hazardous, we should do everything possible to avoid having a child who will have a short or unhappy life. We think that such selectivity provides false comfort, and that such extreme risk aversion is inappropriate both pre- and post-natally—although it clearly has greater costs after birth.

(5) Admittedly, WGS can predict some serious diseases and disabilities a lot better than it can predict mathematical or musical genius. So maybe you can hold the line by testing only for a high probability of one or more conditions on your own list of VSDDs. If you succeed, you'll be in a small minority of the prospective parents who've used PSEDIVG thus far. According to recent research, most demand all the information they can get about the embryos they produce. And most feel felt absolutely overwhelmed and anxious once they receive it. They're staggered by all the uncertainties and choices, and they regret having complicated a process they (believe) used to be simple and joyous. But a surprising proportion don't learn the lesson, going on to test for everything again when they decide to have another child. They apparently suffer from a new kind of pregnancy amnesia.

We used to think that prospective parents would be much less interested in selecting for desirable traits than against disease and disability. As it turns out, we were wrong. One study about a decade ago found that prospective parents seeking ovum donors were increasingly selecting not only for health (72%) but for intelligence (40%) and athletic ability (17%). Now, with PSEDIVG, prospective parents can be their own "donors," but why would they be any less tempted to select for the positive traits to which their own genes contributed?

Of course, you may be the exception to creeping selectivity. But even if you are, even if you can draw a line at VSDDs and hold it, you should ask yourself why you think it's so important to test for even those. Here are a few things to consider:

9.2 Who's Harmed by Not Selecting Against Disease and Disability? Is Anything Wrong with Not Selecting?

(1) You're selecting your future child, not (only) the features your future child will have. Each embryo in the array will, if successfully implanted, become a distinct child, different from any child who would emerge from any other embryo. PSEDIVG cannot make your child happier, healthier, or more successful; it can only select a child expected to be happier, healthier, or more successful than some other child you might have selected. You may prefer that, but don't fool yourself (as some philosophers and bioethicists have) into thinking that you're doing it "for the sake of your child." No actual child will be benefitted by your choice—except in being given a worthwhile existence—and any child you end up with will receive *that* benefit (if it even makes sense to call it a benefit).

(2) Even if you recognize that different embryos mean different children, you may still think it's wrong to choose a child likely to have a VSDD. But first, you need to take the official list with a few grains of salt. Most people with most VSDDs find their lives almost as rich and rewarding as people without VSDDs find theirs. And that's not because they're in denial, or putting up a brave front, or looking on the bright side. You don't need to take their self-appraisals with any more salt than you'd take anyone else's. The simple truth is that there are many ways to live well, and many people with VSDDs have found ways to flourish with them, not despite them. You should also consider the converse: as we've suggested, there are a lot of people with great genetic endowments (and enviable phenotypes) who end up leading miserable lives. You probably know a few. If you don't, we suggest you read the poem "Richard Cory."

(3) You may respectfully disagree with the positive self-assessments of most people with most VSDDs. And, of course, some people with those conditions are far less positive about their lives. Also, most people with certain conditions, especially some psychiatric ones, find their lives even worse than other people think they are. So even if you should resist choosing the happiest or best child, shouldn't you try to minimize the odds of having a child with a really burdensome or disadvantageous condition, even if she will probably be glad to be alive despite having it? Do you have any good reason to pick such a child over one who will not have a known condition that reduces the odds of flourishing? You likely don't, and that's why we don't advise you to select *for* a child with such a condition. Most reasons people would select for such a child, e.g., to give a family member with that condition a close relative to commiserate with—aren't very appealing and suggest that the child is being created "as a mere means." What we advise is that you consider *not selecting at all*. If you end up with a child who has a VSDD, it's still likely to have a good life, and you can give it the best life it can have.

(4) But since, as we've agreed, you have no reason to select such a child, aren't you being insensitive to the hardships of a future child's condition by not selecting against it? After all, it's hardly like you're disfavoring an actual child of yours who has that condition—say, by deciding to give it less time, attention, or resources than its siblings. Unlike children, embryos don't have a right to equal treatment or equal chances. You also don't have any reason to care about one embryo in the array more than another—they're all yours, and you have no basis for individualized attachment.

So why should you give a VSDD embryo any chance, when you could implant an embryo without a VSDD? We'll get to positive reasons for not screening later; for now, we just want to insist that doing so needn't display the slightest insensitivity to its hardships. You would be insensitive if you trivialized those hardships or were indifferent to them. But you could well decline to select against a VSDD even with a keen, realistic appreciation of its hardships. You might, for example, have the condition yourself, and understand both the burdens it imposes and the prospects for living a good life it has given you, or left you with. You might be very glad to be alive, very glad that you had not been screened out. And your gladness might be free of delusion. You might readily agree that you could have had an even better life if you had (somehow) been born without the condition. But that thought would give you no reason to think that your parents would have been insensitive in creating you, if they, like you, had the option of choosing a child without that condition instead.

It's hard to see, then, why you would show the slightest insensitivity if you didn't screen out an embryo with VSDDs, even if you didn't know anyone who had that condition—assuming you took the time to find out what it was like to live with that condition and that you'd be willing and able to give a future child with that condition any extra care that was required. Of course, you don't owe it to an embryo with such a VDSS to implant it, or even to give it a chance of implantation. But you also don't owe it to that embryo *not to*. And you don't owe it to any other embryo, with apparent prospects for an even better life, to implant it instead.

(5) But even if an embryo with a VSDD is likely to have a good life, you may think it would be too painful, burdensome, or expensive *for you* to raise it. If you, your child, or a close family member has grown up with that condition, you're in a pretty good position to make that judgment. But if not, it would be wise to find out about the experiences of parents who have raised children with that condition. You could try to talk with a few, or at least read their blogs. You're likely to find a great deal of variation in their child-rearing experiences and in the lives their children lead. You'll need to weight the evidence you collect. You'll need to ask yourself what kind of life you require or want for yourself and your child, and what kinds of risks and costs you're willing to bear. If you still feel it would be too much for you to raise a child with that condition, it's perfectly reasonable for you to exclude any embryo with it. As we've said, you don't owe the embryo anything.

Thus far, we've urged you to think twice about using PSEDIVG, although we conceded that there are circumstances where it would be reasonable for you to do so. Our main concern has been your own welfare: comprehensive testing is too likely to overload you with information and decisions, and cause high anxiety and bad judgment. We also maintained that it would not be insensitive of you to decline to select against most VSDDs.

We're not done yet, however. First, we want to suggest that there are both moral and prudential reasons to avoid being (too) selective about your future child. Then, shifting gears, we will argue that there are three types of conditions you may have a moral reason to test for: conditions that impose substantial social costs or risk substantial social harms; conditions that are likely to make life not worth living, and conditions that you can prevent, cure, mitigate, or meaningfully prepare for prenatally.

9.3 Are There Moral Reasons Against Prenatal Selectivity?

You might raise your eyebrows at the very idea that you had a moral reason against selectivity. Didn't we just get through saying (several times in fact) that you have no moral obligations to the embryos you produce? We stand by that claim. We recognize that your parental duties towards your children do not extend to your embryos. If you have children that need to be fed, clothed, or housed, you have a duty to feed, clothe, or house all of them. If you tragically can't do so for all of them, it would be gravely wrong to do so only for the children you considered the most talented, kind, loveable, or happy. But, to repeat, you don't have a duty to implant or gestate any of your embryos—you can just drop the parental project and go home. So why should you decline to be selective if you go ahead with it? Our view, which we admit is not widely shared, is that if you decide to proceed, you take on a moral role as a prospective parent, a role that favors an "unconditional welcome" to any embryo you expect to have a decent life.

We don't support this posture because we think it will make you more likely to be unconditionally loving once you become a parent. We agree that having a child can be a transformative experience, and that parents who have been finicky in selecting a child may develop a resilient love for the child they select, even if it acquires conditions more burdensome those some of those they would have selected against. Why, then, do we regard unconditional welcome as an ideal that *prospective* parents should aspire to? It's because we think there's a tension between setting "admission standards" for the kind of children you will have, then completely relinquishing the use of such standards once you have children.

We can illustrate the tension with reference to the sort of imagined dialogue that has been scripted by disability critics of prenatal selection. Consider a condition for which a very accurate genetic test has been recently introduced: severe early-onset asthma. Over 90% of people with specific combinations of genetic variants will develop that condition before the age of 3. You have a 5-year-old child with severe asthma who is doing very well. Sure, the daily vaporizer regime and occasional hospital visits are a hassle—for him and you—but life is full of hassles. The additional effort that his condition requires has become routine; there's so much great about his life that his asthma is little more than an inconvenience.

Shortly after you tell him that you are your spouse are thinking of having another child, he reads about the new test available for severe asthma (He's a precocious reader.) He asks if you are planning to get tested for that condition and why. In fact, despite your happy experience with this child, you've decided that life will be easier for you if you select against that condition in your "next child." You don't want to lie, so you tell your child that you are planning to use the test and avoid having another child with severe asthma. He then asks you if you would have used the test if it were available when you were pregnant with him. You can't be certain, but you're pretty sure you would have, and you tell him that. At the same time, you truthfully assure him that he is the greatest joy in your life and insist, truthfully, that now that he's with you, you do not wish you had done anything differently. He says he believes you, but that it's still painfully clear that you regard his condition as a burden, one that you would have avoided taking on if you could have.

You can't deny this. You can, of course, explain to him that retrospective attitudes are very different than prospective ones. You can tell him that when you were dating, you ruled out obese men. Not only weren't they very appealing to you; you believed that they had shorter life expectancies and you didn't want to spend decades as a widow. Now that you're happily married, however, you wouldn't love your spouse any less if he became obese and prediabetic (even though you'd be concerned about his health). But your precocious child might respond that while that kind of finickiness may be acceptable in dating, it's simply out of placing in starting a family. First, you make an unconditional, lifelong commitment in having a child. Whatever the words of the standard marriage vow, you know you can get divorced, know that almost 50% of all marriages end in divorce, and believe that in many circumstances it's not wrong to divorce. In contrast, while you could put a child up for adoption, it clearly would be wrong to subject a child to the disruption and lasting psychological damage from giving him up, when your only reason for doing so was that he developed a difficult, burdensome health condition.

Second, marriages these days take place among adults. Even if you don't know what fate holds for the two of you, you do know, or should know, a lot about your prospective partner's traits and values. To a large extent, what you see is what you get. In contrast, as we've emphasized, when you have a child, no matter how thoroughly vetted prenatally, you're inviting a stranger into your family, about whom you know and can know very little. It's best, morally and prudentially, for you to embrace this uncertainty from the outset, when you decide whether to test prenatally or what to test for.

Yes, we know you could argue that these differences just reinforce the value of screening: if you're making such a demanding commitment, why not do everything you can to ensure that it's not TOO demanding? Many people have made this opposing argument; however, we believe, and hope we've given you some reason to accept, that such preliminary risk-reduction and burden-lightening are not in the moral spirit of the bold and exiting enterprise you're undertaking.

But wait, didn't we argue a few years back that the state and the reproductive health profession should offer prospective parents information on any traits or predispositions that can be accurately and reliably diagnosed? We did, and that's still our view. We don't think the state should be drawing lines for you, but we think that you should be drawing lines for yourself, very thoughtfully and very narrowly.

We'll conclude with two considerations you should keep in mind when drawing a line: the expected costs of raising a child with a genetically diagnosable condition, and the growing list of genetically-diagnosable conditions that can be prevented, treated, or prepared for prenatally.

9.4 Who Bears the Cost of the Child You're Bearing?

Considerations of cost suggest a qualification of the "unconditional welcome" we've urged you to extend to your future children. Not only should you ask yourselves if you are in a psychological, social, and financial situation to responsibly bear and raise any child, you should ask yourself if you are in a situation where you can responsibly bear and raise a child without imposing extraordinary costs on the state, society, or your parents and siblings.

If it's irresponsible for you to expect third parties to bear most of the costs for you to raise a large number of children, it also may be irresponsible to do so for a single child you expect to be far beyond your psychological, social, or financial means. In both cases, however, claims of irresponsibility need to be viewed with suspicion—they may reflect class, race, ethnic, or disability prejudice, and the state and society may have more responsibility than they are willing to acknowledge in the difficult but critical business of rearing children. We need to view claims about the social costs imposed by women who don't screen against disabilities with the same skepticism we view claims about the social costs imposed by women who don't use contraception when they are on welfare. Both these kinds of "costs" are likely to be vastly exaggerated by bias against the women in question.

Moreover, much or most of the extra cost of raising a child with "special needs" results from injustice and discrimination: in particular, to the failure to build physical structures and social institutions for a wide range of human variation. Concerns about the future productivity of children with disabilities generally ignore the role of exclusionary practices in keeping disabled people unemployed. Much of the additional medical cost of raising disabled children is due to a discriminatory, wasteful, and often dysfunctional healthcare "system." Finally, we suspect that our society is willing to accept much higher costs for many children than for a single child with a disability—compare the joy expressed at the birth of healthy quintuplets with the condolences offered at the birth of a single child with severe cerebral palsy, who will probably have a rewarding life and cost far less to raise.

Still, taking all of this into account, prospective parents bear some responsibility for the costs their procreative decisions impose. It's hardly eugenic to insist that parents should think twice about having children they cannot afford to raise, and who would impose an unfair burden even on an idealized just and efficient society.

9.5 Actionable Results: Therapeutic Testing

We've been insisting that prenatal *selection* can't make your child healthier, but at best give you a different, healthier child. And we're argued that you're not morally required to do that. Prenatal *testing*, however, now gives you an increasing number of ways to make your actual child healthier. Even before the proliferation of fetal therapies we've seen over the past few years, we were able to use prenatal testing to reduce the health risks for some children. For example, we've long known that it's safer to deliver a child with Down syndrome at a hospital with a neonatal cardiovascular ICU, since children with that condition often have cardiac problems requiring immediate attention. For that reason alone, it was worth finding out if your fetus had Trisomy 21. Now, of course, there's more we can do to help a fetus with Down syndrome. Back in 2020, it was demonstrated that by just taking an FDA-approved pill with few side effects, a pregnant woman could increase the neural connectivity in a fetus with Down and thereby mitigate its cognitive impairment. Researchers have just completed successful first -in-human trials of equally safe drugs to prevent or mitigate cardiac problems, and of prenatal laser surgery for more recalcitrant heart defects. And that's just for Down syndrome. We're starting to develop drugs and procedures that may be able to treat dozens of conditions prenatally and significantly reduce the risk of many others.

This all sounds great, until you consider what your pregnancy will be like when all these drugs and procedures become a routine part of prenatal care. You'll soon be facing an array of interventions for diagnosed conditions. Testing for treatable and preventable conditions may require only a single blood draw, but the results are likely to confront you with lots of options and some tough choices. Your fetus will probably be at varying risk for several conditions, for which there will be preventative measures of varying effectiveness, and varying maternal and fetal risks. There's a not-insignificant chance that your fetus will be diagnosed with a condition that can best, or only, be treated with a prenatal intervention that will impose substantial burdens on you.

Remember, if you decide that the drugs have too many nasty side-effects, or that the procedures are too risky or burdensome, you will still have the option of first-trimester abortion (under the latest 5–4 Supreme Court decision). But you wanted this pregnancy. And you want to gestate this fetus. You may have become attached to it; if you're far enough along, you may have felt its movements or heartbeat. How much of a sacrifice are you willing to make to give it the best health modern fetal medicine can provide? Are you willing to settle for less to spare yourself weeks or months of bedrest, risks to future pregnancies, or a non-negligible chance of permanent disability? What if there is uncertainty about the diagnosis, the severity of the condition, or the comparative effectiveness of the interventions? Could you live with yourself if your child developed a serious condition you could or might have prevented by a drug or procedure you declined? Would you feel comfortable telling the child that you weren't willing to make that much of a sacrifice, knowing that it was likely to have a rich and rewarding life even with the diagnosed condition? Would you be willing to mention that you could have aborted, and spared yourself any sacrifices? Or would that not only be tactless and insensitive, but completely improper? Would it be improper to even *consider* the option of abortion in deciding how much prenatal intervention you'd be willing to bear for a wanted child? If the tests you took for "actionable conditions" revealed that your fetus had, or was at risk of developing, a serious condition that you could at best mitigate, not prevent or cure, at substantial personal sacrifice, wouldn't you be tempted to reconsider the whole project? Wouldn't that scintilla of doubt or ambivalence you had about having a child, or having another child, get magnified?

Even if you're willing to make any sacrifice your physician is willing to impose on you, how do you decide what's best for the fetus? The proposed intervention may have significant risks *for it*, from premature delivery to permanent injury and death. You may have to choose between different interventions, for the same or different conditions. Parents often have to make tough decisions about pediatric care, but rarely with the formidable uncertainty, complexity, and time pressure that will face prospective parents balancing fetal and maternal risks.

[Actually, some parents have been facing these tough questions for years. Fetal surgery was pioneered in the 1960s and became more common when prenatal ultrasound was introduced a decade later. In 2010, a major study found that prenatal surgery was significantly more effective than postnatal surgery for treating spina bifida. Since then, hundreds of women have undergone fetal surgery and, doubtless, many have declined—the former are much more likely to blog about their decisions. But now, instead of a few pregnant women facing one difficult choice, many or most will be facing a lot of them.]

Here, unlike in the case of prenatal selection, we don't have much guidance to offer. A woman unwilling to suffer even minor inconvenience or discomfort to protect her future child from a painful, debilitating disease should probably rethink her parental plans, but so should a woman willing to risk her own death or serious injury to remove an unsightly blemish from her fetus. There's a vast space between these extremes, within which reasonable women, and couples, will differ. But we worry that there will be a relentless push toward the latter extreme, as the standards for being "a good mother" prenatally get raised by media celebrations of the heroic sacrifices made by pregnant women to protect their future children. And the increased burden of prenatal care will be borne almost entirely by pregnant women; it's not something their partners can share. Finally, we worry that the devotion of prospective parents to their gestating future children will lead reproductive health professionals, and the public, to regard *all* fetuses, wanted or not, as meriting the same protection. These developments would be at least as disturbing as the anxious, finicky consumerism we've urged you to resist.

9.6 Conclusion

If you think we're giving you mixed messages, we understand. First, we tell you to be very careful about what you test for, emphasizing the risk of confusion, anxiety, and information overload. Then we tell you that you have no moral reason to test for most genetically-based conditions for selection purposes, and maybe perhaps some moral reason not to. But what we discourage with one hand, we seem to demand with the other. There are moral reasons for selecting against some conditions—those "incompatible" with a life worth living, and those that will impose enormous costs on third parties. And there are moral reasons for testing even if you are committed to not selecting—to detect any conditions on the rapidly growing list for which prenatal prevention, treatment, or other action is available. Despite the broader concerns we've raised about fetal medicine, we think that the challenges posed by "therapeutic testing" are ones you should embrace rather than avoid. Conscientious parenting has always been a demanding enterprise, and testing to protect, rather than to select, a future child, strikes us as fully consistent with the evolving role of parents.

Resources for Further Reading

Asch, Adrienne and David Wasserman. 2005. Where is the sin in synecdoche?: prenatal testing and the parent-child relationship. In *Quality of life and human difference: Genetic testing, health care, and disability*, ed. Wasserman, David, Robert Wachbroit, and Jerome Bickenbach. Cambridge: Cambridge University Press.

Bianchi, Diana W. 2012. From prenatal genomic diagnosis to fetal personalized medicine: progress and challenges. *Nature Medicine*, 18 (7): 1041.

Chen, Stephanie C., and David T. Wasserman. 2017. A framework for unrestricted prenatal whole-genome sequencing: Respecting and enhancing the autonomy of prospective parents. *The American Journal of Bioethics* 17 (1): 3–18. [see accompanying Open Peer Commentaries and Response]

Cohen, I. Glenn, George Q. Daley, and Eli Y. Adashi. 2017. Disruptive reproductive technologies. *Science Translational Medicine* 9(372).

Dondorp, Wybo, Guido De Wert, Yvonne Bombard, Diana W. Bianchi, Carsten Bergmann, Pascal Borry, Lyn S. Chitty et al. 2015. Non-invasive prenatal testing for aneuploidy and beyond: challenges of responsible innovation in prenatal screening. *European Journal of Human Genetics* 23 (11): 1438.

Flores, Homero, Joseph Lee, Jorge Rodriguez-Purata, Georgia Witkin, Benjamin Sandler, and Alan B. Copperman. 2014. Beauty, brains or health: Trends in ovum recipient preferences. *Journal of Women's Health* 23 (10): 830–833.

Greely, Henry T. 2018. Human Reproduction in the Twenty-First Century. *Journal of Posthuman Studies* 1 (2): 205–223.

Hendriks, Saskia, Wybo Dondorp, Guido de Wert, Geert Hamer, Sjoerd Repping, and Eline AF Dancet. 2015. Potential consequences of clinical application of artificial gametes: a systematic review of stakeholder views. *Human Reproduction Update* 21 (3): 297–309.

Lyerly, Anne Drapkin, Elena A. Gates, Robert C. Cefalo, and Jeremy Sugarman. 2001. Toward the ethical evaluation and use of maternal-fetal surgery." *Obstetrics & Gynecology* 98 (4): 689–697.

Minear, Mollie A., Stephanie Alessi, Megan Allyse, Marsha Michie, and Subhashini Chandrasekharan. 2015. Noninvasive prenatal genetic testing: Current and emerging ethical, legal, and social issues. *Annual Review of Genomics and Human Genetics* 16: 369–398.

Wasserman, David. 2015. Disability Perspectives. In *Prenatal and Preimplantation Diagnosis*, 229–245. Cham: Springer.

Wasserman, David. 2018. Fetal Medicine and the Pregnant Woman. *Hastings Center Report* 48 (2): inside-back.

Index

M. A. Allyse and M. Michie (eds.), *Born Well: Prenatal Genetics and the Future of Having Children*, The International Library of Bioethics 88,
https://doi.org/10.1007/978-3-030-82536-2

The manufacturer's authorised representative in the EU is Springer Nature Customer Service Centre GmbH, Europaplatz 3, 69115 Heidelberg, Germany. If you have any concerns regarding our products, please contact ProductSafety@springernature.com

Printed and bound by CPI Group (UK) Ltd, Croydon, CR0 4YY
28/09/2026
02224086-0017